Essay Plans for Anaesthesia Exams

For Churchill Livingstone
Publisher: Simon Fathers
Project Editor: Clare Wood-Allum
Editorial Co-ordination: Editorial Resources Unit
  Copy Editor: Andrew Gardiner
Production Controller: Neil Dickson
Design: Design Resources Unit
Sales Promotion Executive: Caroline Boyd

Essay Plans for Anaesthesia Exams

Maher Z. Michel MB ChB MS FCAnaes
Senior Registrar in Anaesthesia, Department of Anaesthesia, Southampton
General Hospital, Southampton, UK; Currently Acting Assistant Professor, Department
of Anesthesiology, University of Washington, Seattle, Washington, USA

Neville W. Goodman MA(Oxon) DPhil BM BCh FCAnaes
Consultant Senior Lecturer in Anaesthesia, University of Bristol
and Southmead Hospital, Bristol, UK

Alan R. Aitkenhead BSc MD FCAnaes
Professor of Anaesthesia, University of Nottingham, Department of Anaesthesia, Queen's
Medical Centre, Nottingham, UK

CHURCHILL LIVINGSTONE
EDINBURGH LONDON MADRID MELBOURNE NEW YORK AND TOKYO 1992

CHURCHILL LIVINGSTONE
Medical Division of Longman Group UK Limited

Distributed in the United States of America by Churchill
Livingstone Inc., 650 Avenue of the Americas, New York, N.Y. 10011,
and by associated companies, branches and representatives throughout the world.

First published 1992

ISBN 0-443-04395-7

British Library of Cataloguing in Publication Data
A catalogue record for this book is available from the British Library.

Library of Congress Cataloging in Publication Data
A catalog record for this book is available from the Library of Congress.

The
publisher's
policy is to use
paper manufactured
from sustainable forests

Produced by Longman Singapore Publishers (Pte) Ltd
Printed in Singapore

Preface

This book is intended for candidates preparing for Part 1 or Part 3 of the FCAnaes examination. Its origins lie in the preparations for the Part 3 examination by one of the authors, who realised that it might improve his performance to prepare logical plans as answers to previous, and predicted, essay questions. His original comprehensive essay plans have been reviewed, summarised and annotated, with the purpose of presenting a logical framework from which essays on common topics can be constructed.

There are two basic requirements for success in an examination: possession of knowledge, and the ability to demonstrate that knowledge to the examiners. Textbooks, journals and senior colleagues are the sources of knowledge and understanding. Some candidates fail examinations through lack of knowledge, but many fail because their answers are misdirected or lack structure and the examiner is left unaware of the candidate's learning or comprehension of the subject.

The book is not intended to provide short notes for revision. It is not intended to act as an aide-memoire. It does not provide the answers to essay questions. Its purposes are to help the candidate to analyse the important parts of a question, to differentiate the relevant subject matter from the irrelevant, to divide the topic up into appropriate segments, and to apportion discussion of each topic rationally. In addition, we have tried to point out potential traps and common mistakes to which candidates often succumb. The questions are divided into sections so that candidates can use the book during revision. Although many of the questions are similar to those that have appeared in FCAnaes examinations, we have not attempted to provide a comprehensive list; new topics arise, and the emphasis of a question may be changed significantly by rewording. However, we believe that there are new lessons to be learnt from each of the 75 questions. We hope that by constructing essay plans for these questions, and by comparing their plans with the suggestions contained in the book, the candidate will be helped in revision, and will develop the ability to answer essay questions in a logical and structured manner to ensure that the examiner is made fully aware of the knowledge and understanding that the candidate has acquired from other sources.

Southampton, Bristol and Nottingham 1992   M.Z.M.
N.W.G.
A.R.A.

Contents

CHAPTER 3 **Physics, measurement and equipment**

CHAPTER 4 **General anaesthesia**

CHAPTER 5 **Anaesthesia for specific diseases or conditions**

Introduction: how to use this book

To pass an examination you must have knowledge and you must be able to present it. This book provides some advice on where to acquire the knowledge, but its main function is to test whether candidates are able to structure that knowledge efficiently and impress the examiners with an understanding of the subjects about which they are writing.

There are many textbooks about anaesthesia but it is difficult to use them to assess attempted essay questions. The most obvious reason for this is that the books contain too much detail, but there is another, more subtle, reason. Candidates certainly fail essay questions because they do not know enough facts, but they also fail commonly because their essays have poor structure. By failing to use a sensible structure, candidates fail to show they understand the relative importance of parts of the answer, and sometimes leave out important sections entirely.

The reading must come before the planning. For Part 1 of the examination, the new Diploma (DA), the standard textbooks alone will be enough; for Part 3 of the examination, your reading will have to be wider.

There are many standard textbooks, and no single one can be picked out as 'the best'. It is probably true that books based on British practice are better when preparing for the British examinations. Textbooks are personal things and, if you like the look and feel of a book, that is a good reason for using it. All textbooks contain some errors, but none contains so many that use of it for an examination will risk candidates' failing. Some people like short textbooks, which supply just about everything they need to know; other people prefer a longer book, from which they can be selective in their reading. For Part 1, the less specialized books, perhaps a 'compendium' textbook that contains chapters on just about everything, are best for most people.

Even in your first year in the specialty of anaesthesia, particularly if you intend to make the specialty your career, you should do some reading beyond the textbooks. Innovation, originality and topicality lend interest to any subject, and they are not usually found in textbooks. The easiest journal is *Anaesthesia*, and you should look at the editorials and review articles. At this early stage, do not forget journals that have occasional reviews of anaesthetic interest, such as the *British Journal of Hospital Medicine*.

Once you decide that you are a career anaesthetist, and have passed Parts 1 and 2, you should get into the firm habit of reading editorials in the leading journals: *Anaesthesia, British Journal of Anaesthesia, Anesthesia and Analgesia* and *Anesthesiology*. Editorials show what is topical, and give a current expert opinion. They often supply a succinct answer to an essay question in a way that a textbook rarely can. You should consider editorials from the three years up to the time of the examination; and study the ones from the immediately preceding 12 months particularly well — the examiners will have read them recently too!

Reviews in these four journals can bring what you have read in the textbooks more up to date, or may mean that you can skip that chapter in the book. The *Canadian Journal of Anesthesia* and the *European Journal of Anaesthesiology* also publish review articles. There are review journals as well, but a good habit of keeping up with the standard journals will keep you up to date. Do not forget to glance at the *British Medical Journal* and the *Lancet*; you are a doctor first and an anaesthetist second.

There are many other journals — the *New England Journal of Medicine* is one of the best from North America — and, in your preparation for the Part 3, there are many specialized monographs and also books that are collections of reviews. You must realize early on that it is simply impossible to read everything; the key to sensible learning is sensibly selective reading.

Assuming you have assimilated a reasonable amount of information, you now need a strategy to get it down on paper in the 25 to 35 minutes allotted to each answer. There are two things you must do.

1. Take time to think and make a plan.
2. Answer the question.

The plan should take a full five minutes per half hour allotted. Use a full page of the answer book — or more if you need it — to write headings, rough out diagrams, and jot down key words. Write numbers by the headings in order of importance. Use underlining and asterisks. Do not worry if people around you are scribbling furiously; if your thoughts are ordered, you will have plenty of time in which to write a full answer.

While making your plan, bear the second point in mind all the time: answer the question. If the question is 'Describe two methods of performing local analgesia of the brachial plexus' then you will gain nothing from describing three methods. If the question is 'What are the features of a ventilator that makes it suitable for use in the intensive care unit?' then you will gain nothing from a description of ventilators suited to the operating theatre, no matter how correct.

Helping you to draw up a plan for essay questions is the main aim of this book. In fact, it is possible to write a basic essay plan for a subject about which you know nothing. Even if you have no idea of what plate tectonics is (it is the theory of drifting continents) it is possible to make a plan for an essay on the effect of plate tectonics on the British landscape:

Definition of plate tectonics
Britain's basic structure
How plate tectonics has altered Britain in the past
Effects of plate tectonics happening today
How plate tectonics may affect Britain in the future

Without further knowledge, that is as far as you will get; but the basic outline is there. You may be unfortunate enough in the examination to have to answer a question about which you know little, but the discipline of making essay plans will at least give you the best chance of salvaging the situation.

At the time of writing there is no choice in Part 1; there are seven compulsory questions. In Part 3, there are two sections of four questions each. Five questions have to be answered, at least two from each section. Some candidates prefer to sketch out all their plans before starting any definitive answers; this has the advantage that if thoughts for one of the other questions occur to you during the writing of an answer, you can add them to the appropriate plan. Others write plans before each definitive answer. Whichever you prefer, write your best answer first because it gives you longer to think about your weaker answers. After each answer is written, make a cross through the plan so the examiners cannot mistake it for your answer. Do not spend too long on the first two or three answers; running out of time is a foolish way of failing an examination. In an examination you must work to the clock.

The plan for a question on a particular topic is likely to be much the same whatever the wording of the question, but the method of expansion will depend on whether the question asks you to 'Describe . . .', 'Discuss . . .', 'Write short notes on . . .', and so on. An examination consisting of essay questions demands answers that are written in sentences organized into paragraphs. Even a question worded 'Write short notes on . . .' must be answered in a logical way.

Write neatly and legibly. Use headings and underlining, but sparingly, to draw the examiners' attention to the key points. Even though the examiners will not be deducting marks for grammatical errors, you should try to write simple, plain language. Do not be tempted to waffle as a way of disguising lack of knowledge; examiners see through it.

It is better to avoid using abbreviations but, if you do use them, use only standard ones, and always define them when first used. Use abbreviations only for phrases that you will be writing repeatedly, not for phrases that you will be writing only once or twice. In the question 'What are the uses of capnography in the operating theatre?' the use of the standard abbreviations $PaCO_2$, $PACO_2$, and $PE'CO_2$ would be acceptable. However, in the question 'Describe the insertion of a flow-directed pulmonary artery catheter and list some indices of cardiac performance that the catheter could be used to measure', a list of abbreviations would not be satisfactory.

Never use abbreviations simply as shorthand. No matter how many times you need to write *epidural* in the question 'Write an essay about the management of pain in normal labour', it should not be shortened to, for example, EPI or E. People who are keen on writing abbreviations complain that otherwise they do not have time to answer the questions, but this is a false argument. Any question set in the FCAnaes examinations can be answered in the allotted time by writing slowly and carefully. You are not being asked to write everything you know about a subject; you are being asked to organize your knowledge so that you present to the examiner an appropriate amount of detail. After all, there are whole books about obstetric anaesthesia, and you cannot write a book in 35 minutes.

If the question can be answered with a diagram, make it large and clear. Use a ruler to draw straight lines. Colour can help, but cannot be rubbed out as easily as ordinary pencil, so pencil is better if you are not certain of getting everything correct first time. There is no need for the writing to repeat what is obvious from the diagram, and for some questions an annotated diagram may be all that is needed.

There is probably little significance in the exact form of wording of a question. Whether the question starts 'Describe . . .', 'Discuss . . .', or 'Compare and contrast . . .' your answer is likely to be the same; most of these differences in wording are only for variety and you can take them all to mean 'Write an essay on . . .'.

The first steps to answering a question, and therefore to making the plan, are reading the question, writing it out on the answer sheet, and underlining the key words.

Q   1.0   Write an essay about the management of pain in normal labour.

Here the key words are *pain* and *normal*. This question does not include anaesthesia for delivery by forceps, or Caesarean section, and underlining *normal* helps to imprint this.

There are then three basic structures that are always worth remembering: physiology — altered physiology — pathology; preop — perop (induction — maintenance — immediate recovery) — postop; discovery — development — current practice — the future. There are few questions for which some of this structure does not apply. The opening section of your answer is very important; it is a base for development. In the question on pain in labour, the base is the physiology: start with a brief summary of where, why and when the pain is felt in the stages of labour.

How should the subject of pain relief then be introduced? It is very easy at this point to assume that the question is asking about epidural analgesia, because epidural analgesia is the most important aspect for the anaesthetist. Almost certainly, candidates who make this interpretation will fail, although the answer should probably have more detail about epidural analgesia than other methods. The answer should continue with the other methods, using something of the *discovery — development — current practice* line.

A word or two about Simpson, Snow and chloroform could be put in here. Nitrous oxide follows logically, and deserves expansion because it is used widely. Finish the section with a comment about methoxyflurane and trichloroethylene.

Next come systemic analgesics, and a discussion of the uses and problems of (mainly) pethidine. This necessitates some discussion of the placental transfer of drugs, which you can follow up in the next section, the most important part of the answer, about epidural analgesia.

This is a question about general management, not specific technique. With all the other topics that have to be included, there will not be time to write about the details of how you do an epidural; mention of the need for intravenous infusion, aseptic technique and identification of the space will be enough. A question asking 'Describe a technique for insertion of an epidural catheter for relief of pain in labour' would require descriptions of volumes of fluid, preparation of the patient, testing of equipment, and so on. (On the other hand, writing about Snow or pethidine would not now be required.)

Lastly, do not forget transcutaneous nerve stimulation, breathing exercises and psychological support. Remember also that some women do not use, need, or want relief of pain.

What you might have on your answer paper by this time, though perhaps in a more shorthand style, would be:

Write an essay about the management of <u>pain</u> in <u>normal labour</u>.

Physiology:
 first stage
  pathways ?diagram
 second stage
  pathways

History: Simpson, chloroform

Nitrous oxide: Entonox, demand valve (safety)
 rapid on/off
 physiological effects (esp hyperventilation)

mental state
lack of fetal effect

Other inhalational agents

Pethidine: best early

disadvantages
including drowsiness, placental transfer

Epidural: informed consent, IVI

insertion of catheter, test dose, dosage scheme
main side-effects (mention of spinal headache)
operative procedures
Other: TENS, psychological

This is the format of the plans that form the main part of this book. The items that should appear in the plans will be inset. Any comments that we make about sections of the plan will follow those sections and be printed across the full width of the page, as below. Often, comments will be warnings of what should *not* be included in the answer.

[In the plan:]

Pethidine: best early

disadvantages
including drowsiness, placental transfer

[Our comment:]

Do not be disparaging about pethidine. Although it has disadvantages, there are many obstetric units where epidural services cannot be provided.

There is no single correct answer to any question, which means there is no single correct plan. For some questions in the book we give suggestions for a different structure. Your plan may progress differently, but as long as it progresses logically it should enable a good answer. Discuss your suggested plan with colleagues and compare your plans with our suggestions. Discuss them with your consultant and senior registrar colleagues. There is a tendency before examinations for candidates to disappear into the library and attempt to read everything in sight, but discussion of issues with colleagues is one of the most valuable forms of preparation. Particularly at Part 3, questions may require an opinion based on considered evidence, and discussions of points of view will help you frame arguments.

One other feature of the plans in the book is that we give suggested opening sentences. The opening sentence of an essay is the most important one: it allows you to show the examiners that you understand the question, and that you understand why it was asked. Examiners are human; if they see a clearly laid-out plan and read a clear, apposite, first sentence, they are likely to be kindly inclined towards you.

Good opening sentences for the example question would be:

> Pain in the first stage of labour is felt in the lower thoracic and upper lumbar segments, and in the second stage is felt also in the sacral segments.

> There are three common methods of relieving pain in labour: pethidine injections, Entonox inhalation, and epidural analgesia.

> Pain during labour was thought by many to be essential to the health of the mother and baby until Queen Victoria accepted John Snow's chloroform.

These opening sentences are, respectively, physiological, summary, and historical. Beware of simply restating the question or writing something that is self-evident.

> There are many ways of providing pain relief in labour.

> Anaesthetists have a major role to play in providing pain relief to labouring mothers.

Both these statements are true, but they are padding.

The 75 questions in the book are listed on pages vii–xi. The suggested plans follow on pages 9–187, arranged in Chapters under broad subject headings. There are two ways of approaching the questions: either attempt a specific Chapter after you have revised its subject; or choose a number, say three, questions at random. Answer your chosen questions unseen, taking the full five minutes for each plan.

Whatever approach you use, you will gain little from looking at a plan before attempting one of your own. Each question has an Outline Plan, so that you can check quickly that your plan covers the broad headings. If your logical sequence is different from ours, the Outline Plan should allow you to orientate yourself as you read through the detailed plan and comments. For the question discussed on the previous pages, the Outline Plan would be:

> **Physiology**: stages, pathways
> **History**
> **Nitrous oxide**: equipment, pharmacology
> **Pethidine**
> **Epidural**: informed consent, technique
>   doses, side-effects
> **Other**

Some Outline Plans, which might otherwise be rather non-specific, contain more detail.

The questions are similar to those asked in the Part 1 and Part 3 examinations of the FCAnaes in the last few years. All questions are appropriate at Part 3. Some are too specialized for Part 1. Where a question is appropriate for both Parts of the examination, it is obvious that a deeper level of knowledge and understanding will be required at Part 3 and sometimes we have indicated these areas of knowledge in the plans. Equally obviously, we cannot do this extensively for all plans; that is what the textbooks and discussions with your tutors and colleagues are for.

Finally, the plan is important, but it is not the definitive answer. Write a few full answers before the examination and ask senior colleagues to read them. Only by doing this will you be able to practise timing yourself properly in preparation for the examination hall.

CHAPTER 1

Anatomy and regional analgesia

INTRODUCTION

Anatomical questions are fairly stereotyped. They are often in two parts, the first being straightforward anatomy, the second an applied aspect of that anatomy. These questions are a test of two types of knowledge: theoretical knowledge derived from reading textbooks of anatomy and practical knowledge derived from clinical experience. There is no better way of knowing how to describe an axillary block clearly, sensibly and succinctly than by doing 30 of them before you sit the Part 3 examination. However, although this experience will teach you the problems and pitfalls of the block, it will not teach you the relation between nerve roots and peripheral nerves.

Anatomical questions are a gift to those who have done the work. They require little thought or organization at the time because the organization is inherent in the knowledge — not always so for the more complex clinical questions. However, you will fail the question if you do not satisfy the examiner in both parts: describing all the tricks for a successful ankle block will not encourage leniency in the examiner if you show that you simply have no idea which nerve comes from where. However, do not worry if you cannot remember the smaller details of anatomy.

Always draw a diagram if appropriate (see p. 4). Anatomical questions commonly do not need an opening sentence, particularly if you draw a large, clear diagram on the first page of the answer book. Diagrams suitable for answers are best developed yourself from a standard textbook. Textbooks of anatomy usually have the clearest diagrams but too much detail. Working with both an anaesthetic textbook and an anatomy textbook can be helpful. Alternatively, there are textbooks of anaesthetic anatomy and of techniques of local anaesthesia.

The plans for the anatomical parts of these questions list only the most important branches or structures.

1–1 Describe the sensory innervation of the lower limb. How would you undertake ankle block for surgery of the foot?

OUTLINE PLAN

Lumbar plexus

iliohypogastric, ilioinguinal, genitofemoral,

lateral cutaneous nerve of thigh
posterior branch of femoral nerve
obturator

Sacral plexus

posterior cut nv thigh
sciatic nerve
  tibial nerve:
  common peroneal nerve:
perforating cutaneous branches

Ankle block: GA?, patient, preparation, solutions

nerves and injections

The lower limb extends anteriorly to the groin crease and includes the buttocks posteriorly. There is no need to write this because your diagram will show it. The origins of each named sensory nerve can be shown by different colours in your diagram, or you can give a list. This part of the question is answered satisfactorily by a list, the skeleton for which is given here.

If you want an opening sentence:

Sensory innervation of the lower limb is by branches of the lumbar and sacral plexuses.

Diagrams

Lumbar

iliohypogastric (L1)
ilioinguinal (L1)
genitofemoral (L1,2)
lateral cutaneous nerve of thigh (L2,3)
femoral nerve (L2,3,4):
  posterior branch:
    medial cut nv of thigh
    intermediate cut nv of thigh
    saphenous
obturator (L2,3,4) : (NB knee)

The question asks for sensory innervation, and is mostly about cutaneous sensation. Do not forget the joints. A comment is appropriate here because of the practical difficulties of blocking the obturator nerve for operations on the knee.

Sacral

posterior cut nv of thigh (S1,2,3)
sciatic nerve (L4,5 and S1,2,3):
  tibial nerve:
    sural
    medial and lateral plantar

> medial calcaneal
> common peroneal nerve:
>   lateral cut nv of calf
>   deep peroneal nerve
>   superficial peroneal nerve
> Perforating cutaneous branches (S2,3)

You may have learned the alternative nomenclature, by which the tibial is the medial popliteal, and becomes the posterior tibial when the lateral popliteal — otherwise the common peroneal — separates. The deep peroneal is the anterior tibial; the superficial peroneal the musculocutaneous. These alternative names are confusing but try not to mix the two nomenclatures.

Describing the anatomy should take half the allotted time. The question then asks *How would you undertake ankle block for surgery of the foot?* This makes it a general question; it does not ask specifically about an operation for hallux valgus or amputation of the forefoot. In your answer you can give examples of when it is particularly important that one or other nerve is blocked effectively. Five nerves have to be blocked, but the answer needs more than just a list of those nerves and how you approach them.

Ankle block

> with or without GA: approach patient
> preparation: of room, of patient
> solution: dose, vasoconstrictor

If the question asked *Which nerves need to be blocked...?* then there would be no need for this introductory section. Phrased as it is, the question demands it. An ankle block in an awake patient may be the best approach, but it requires skill, patience and a willing patient. You do not need detail of the necessary preparations (resuscitation equipment and intravenous access) nor is it necessary to describe preoperative assessment of the patient.

Then for each nerve, you need the surface marking, the approach, and the volume of solution. There is no substitute for experience, and this book is even less suitable than a textbook of local anaesthesia for 'learning' the technique.

Nerves

> posterior tibial
> saphenous nerve
> superficial peroneal nerve/musculocutaneous
> deep peroneal nerve/anterior tibial
> sural nerve

Injections

> behind medial malleolus
> between tendons anteriorly then extend

subcutaneously medially and laterally
subcutaneously posteriorly from lateral malleolus

1-2 Describe the anatomy of the caudal (sacral) epidural space. Discuss the indications for epidural block performed by the caudal route.

OUTLINE PLAN

Anatomy
relations
superiorly, inferiorly, anteriorly, posteriorly, laterally
contents
sacral hiatus
volume

Indications
paediatrics
perineal operations in adults
obstetrics
other:
surgery
pain clinic

The caudal space is a three-dimensional space and it is not easy to draw a clear diagram. By all means draw one, but the caudal space can be described in words quite well if you think in standard anatomical terms.

The caudal epidural space is a cavity of triangular cross-section running the length of the sacrum.

Superiorly: lumbar vertebral canal

Inferiorly: sacral hiatus

Anteriorly: vertebral bodies

Posteriorly: laminae

Laterally: anterior and posterior sacral foraminae

Contents
dural sac, filum terminale
sacral nerve roots, coccygeal nerve root
venous plexus
areolar and fatty tissues
fibrous strands

Anaesthetic anatomy is usually asked with an applied motive. The motive here is explicit (caudal block) but, even if it had not been, the most important aspect of the anatomy of this region is the sacral hiatus, which allows anaesthetists access to the space. Some detail of this is needed even if the question asks only for the anatomy.

Sacral hiatus

triangular opening, missing 5th (4th) laminar arch
sacral cornua
sacrococcygeal membrane (S5 and coccygeal nerve)

Volume: 34 ml (adult male) BUT variable leakage

The second part of the question is worded precisely: 'Discuss the *indications* for epidural block performed by the caudal route'. It asks only for indications, not for method, choice of drug, dosage or complications. These aspects should be mentioned only if they have a bearing on the indication (for example, if a possible indication requires close to the maximum permitted dose).

Start with a general statement about the difficulties of predicting effect because of variable leakage through the foramina. The uses are then probably best discussed under the headings paediatrics, perineal operations in adults, obstetrics, and other.

Paediatrics

technically simple, reliable, effective
relatively safe
especially circumcision, hernia repair

Perineal operations in adults

anatomy not so easy in adults
especially haemorrhoidectomy
especially 'one-shot' combined with GA

Obstetrics

forceps delivery
pain relief after episiotomy
continuous caudal for pain relief during labour

If you work in a unit where continuous caudals are used then describe some of the advantages and disadvantages. Nowadays, lumbar epidurals are far more common, and anaesthetic examinations are about clinical practice. The main advantage is the excellent perineal analgesia; the main disadvantage is the increased risk of infection and the oft-quoted and usually remembered risk of puncture of the fetal head.

Other

surgery to lower limb
transurethral operations
therapeutic indications (pain clinic)

Given the ready availability now of fine spinal needles, there are few anaesthetists who would prefer to give a caudal to a spinal (subarachnoid) anaesthetic for operations on the leg or for a transurethral procedure.

1-3   Describe the anatomy of the inguinal canal. Discuss techniques for local anaesthesia for herniorrhaphy excluding extradural and subarachnoid block.

OUTLINE PLAN

Internal and external rings

Walls of canal

Contents

spermatic cord/round ligament
  contents
ilio-inguinal nerve

Innervation

courses and areas supplied

Indications and contraindications

Field block by three weals

Infiltration technique

Supplementation

The examiner wants to know that you understand the anatomy of the inguinal canal well enough to provide local anaesthesia, not well enough to repair a hernia. Diagrams, if not drawn carefully, may be more confusing than a written description and diagrams alone are unlikely to be sufficient.

The opening sentence should take you straight into the anatomical description.

The inguinal canal is 4 cm long in the adult, lying above the medial half of the inguinal ligament, and extending laterally from the internal ring to the external ring.

Internal and external ring: muscle and surface marking

walls of canal
  anterior, posterior, floor and roof

Contents

spermatic cord/round ligament
  vas deferens
  arteries
  veins and lymphatics

> autonomic fibres
> ilio-inguinal nerve

With more detail, that should suffice for anatomical description. The second part of the question asks you to 'Discuss techniques . . . for herniorrhaphy . . .', and is easiest to answer logically if in the next section you describe the nerve supply to the area. A diagram may help here.

Course and area supplied: (diagram)

> T11 and T12 segmental nerves
> iliohypogastric nerve
> ilio-inguinal nerve
> genitofemoral nerve
> > genital and femoral branches

There are really only two techniques of local anaesthesia: field block and infiltration. Start this section with some discussion of when a local technique is indicated, and then describe the two techniques.

Indications and contraindications

> patient factors, hernia factors, surgeon factors

Field block

> three weals
> 1. for external oblique aponeurosis
> 2. pubis
> 3. above ligament

Infiltration technique

Anyone who has done a field block will recognize the shorthand description. Placement of needle and dose of drug must be given for each site. This book is not the place for more detail. Anyone with experience of the block will also know that supplementation may be necessary.

Supplementation

> along incision
> at ring
> deeper layers
> femoral hernia

Infiltration technique

The question specifically excludes extradural and subarachnoid anaesthesia, but you would be surprised how many candidates will want to write a sentence or two 'just for completeness'. Do not do that; the question is complete without peridural anaesthesia (which includes paravertebral block). It *is* worth discussing the efficacy of local anaesthesia as sole anaesthetic, the advantages of the technique (which include that there is no need for an anaesthetist if the surgeon is skilled in local anaesthesia), and (briefly) their use combined with a general anaesthetic.

1-4   Describe the anatomy of the diaphragm. Discuss the factors encountered in anaesthetic practice which affect the function of the diaphragm.

OUTLINE PLAN

Origins and attachments
  crura & arcuate ligaments
  costal & xiphoid

Structures passing through
  inferior vena cava
  oesophagus, vagi
  aorta, azygos vein, thoracic duct
  others

Nerve supply
  motor & sensory

Function
  ventilation
  raising intra-abdominal pressure
  lower oesophageal sphincter

Changes
  at induction
  with neuromuscular relaxation

Posture

Abdominal splinting

The anatomy of the diaphragm includes its origin and insertions, the structures (vessels, viscus, nerves) that pass through it, and the structures that pass behind it (vessels, nerves, muscles). There is no better way to describe this than by diagrams. You could precede the diagrams with a sentence or two of general description.

The diaphragm, the most important muscle of ventilation, forms a musculotendinous partition between the thoracic and abdominal cavities, through which pass the aorta, inferior vena cava, oesophagus, and other structures.

Your plan should be either a rough sketch or a list — probably both, otherwise you are likely to forget things that are difficult to represent in diagrams, such as the sensory nerve supply.

Origins and attachments
  crura: left and right
  arcuate ligaments: median, medial, lateral
  costal
  xiphoid

Structures passing through

> inferior vena cava
> oesophagus, vagi
> aorta, azygos vein, thoracic duct
> others

Nerve supply:

> motor
> sensory

You may well not remember all the structures passing through the diaphragm while you are writing the plan. Once you have started on the diagrams for the full answer, jot structures down as they occur to you — they include important structures such as the sympathetic trunk and the splanchnic nerves. Annotate your diagrams in some detail, expanding the labels to give information, e.g. 'Central tendon (continuous with fibrous pericardium above)' and 'Phrenic nerve (C3,4,5)'. This is quicker and less awkward than giving descriptions in words.

The second part of the question is the effect of 'anaesthetic factors' (an odd way of phrasing the question) on function. Recall the basic structures for answers (see p. 5): physiology — altered physiology. Do not launch off into this part with 'When a patient is anaesthetized . . .'; describe the normal function first.

Function

> ventilation
> raising intra-abdominal pressure
> lower oesophageal sphincter

Everyone will know of the importance of the diaphragm in breathing and the prevention of regurgitation; its importance in raising intra-abdominal pressure during defecation, micturition, vomiting and giving birth may be forgotten.

You may choose to discuss the effects of anaesthetic factors after each heading of normal function or as a separate section. Whichever is your approach you must discuss:

Changes

> at induction
> with neuromuscular relaxation

Posture

Abdominal splinting

The changes are mostly of the relative movements of different parts of the diaphragm, which does not move as a single muscle. Discuss these changes and their effect on ventilation/perfusion ratio.

1-5   Describe the anatomy of the first rib. Outline the technique of infraclavicular subclavian vein catheterization.

OUTLINE PLAN

Features
head
neck & tubercle
superior surface
markings
inner margin
outer margin

Catheterization
patient
operator
site
equipment
procedure:
needle direction
successful puncture
action if unsuccessful
guide wire, catheter
fixation
checking

Some diagrams, for instance of the diaphragm or the brachial plexus, are easy to draw. The first rib is not easy to draw, but you are being given marks for knowledge not for artistic ability. Do not worry if the scale of your diagram is incorrect as long as you have indicated the relative positions of the various marks and grooves on the bone, *but lack of artistic ability is no excuse for untidiness.*

Start your answer simply with your diagrams, or with a short introduction.

The first rib is the shortest and flattest rib.

Features
head with facet
neck, tubercle (transverse process of T1)
crossed by: sympathetic trunk
first thoracic nerve
superior intercostal artery
superior surface
scalenus medius
subclavian artery, brachial plexus
scalene tubercle

subclavian vein
origin of subclavius muscle
inner margin: Sibson's fascia
outer margin: muscular attachments

You are asked for an *outline* of the technique of the *infraclavicular* approach. You do not need to discuss the indications or the general preparations. *Do not* mention the supraclavicular approach, or the low approach to the internal jugular vein, even to compare their ease of use or safety.

Your full answer must describe a logical sequence, so take time getting your plan correct: the examiners will not be impressed by an answer in which you insert the needle before you remember to position the patient.

Patient: basic position, comfort

Operator: sterility

Site: identify, infiltrate, drape

Equipment

Procedure: fine position
re-identify
needle direction
successful puncture
unsuccessful: no blood
arterial blood
air or cough
guide wire, then catheter
fixation
checking

The basic position is head down; 'fine position' means the position of the patient's head and ipsilateral arm. 'Comfort' is important; the patient who is awake should be able to talk to a nurse, who can also help to keep the drapes away from the face.

Describe the equipment first in a general way — for instance syringe size, needle gauge, and guide wire — and second mention any commercially available kit with which you are familiar.

You must describe the direction of puncture clearly. Some people develop tricks, such as putting a slight bend on the needle so that the syringe is not pushed anteriorly by the shoulder. Put these in your answer if they have helped you in your practice. Your answer must include the correct action in the event of incorrect puncture.

The method of fixation depends on the indication for the catheter (for example, a simple adhesive occlusive dressing in the short term or a tunnelled line for parenteral nutrition); a short discussion is better than a simple statement that the catheter must be sutured to the skin.

1-6 Describe the anatomy of the eighth intercostal nerve. Discuss the indications and methods for performing an intercostal nerve block. What complications may occur?

OUTLINE PLAN

Anatomy

    sketch

Intercostal block

    indications

        perioperative

        fractured ribs

        (contraindications)

    standard method

        approaches

        technique

    direct vision

        cryoanalgesia

    complications

        puncture of blood vessels

        pneumothorax

        hypotension

        overdosage

The obvious opening sentence is perfectly good.

The eighth intercostal nerve is the anterior primary ramus of T8.

It is probably worth writing a couple of sentences describing the relation of the nerve to the muscles as it passes anteriorly, and another sentence summarizing the innervation. The first section of the question can be answered completely by diagrams (and you should check your knowledge of the anatomy against diagrams in the textbooks).

Intercostal block

    indications

        postoperative pain relief

        operative: abdominal

          rib resection

        fractured ribs

        (contraindications)

Antibiotics have reduced the incidence of empyema needing operative drainage but the procedure is still in the books. The contraindications are general to the use of local anaesthetics rather than specific to the technique.

        standard method

approaches: posterior, midaxillary
technique
    site, needle size, identification
drug and dose
catheter
direct vision
    local anaesthetic solution
    cryoanalgesia using cryoprobe

Complications

puncture of blood vessels
pneumothorax
hypotension
overdosage

Discussion of the complications includes management of them. Hypotension can occur if local anaesthetic solution spreads to the paravertebral, or even epidural, space. The theoretical motor weakness that is caused by paralysis of intercostal muscles is probably not worth mentioning.

This is the sort of question that should be easy to pass, which is another way of saying that it is mainly concerned with facts and not very exciting.

1-7 Discuss the prevention and treatment of the main complications of epidural analgesia using local anaesthetic drugs.

OUTLINE PLAN

Hypotension

Dural tap

Unblocked segment, unilateral block

Effects of drug overdose

Paraesthesia

Extradural haematoma

Infection

The question asks about epidural analgesia: do not misread the question as asking about spinal analgesia (see the next question). Do not include any discussion of peridural opioids.

In the first sentence, one approach is to emphasize those complications you deem the most important and that you will be discussing at greatest length.

The most important complications of an epidural injection of local anaesthetic are hypotension and the risk of overdose of the drug.

Although there are a number of important and potentially dangerous complications of epidural analgesia, the complications that often cause most difficulty to the anaesthetist, especially in obstetric practice, are the benign but frustrating ones of missed segments and unilateral block, and the distressing problem of dural tap.

Another approach is to make a general statement.

Most of the complications of epidural analgesia can be prevented, or at least their effects made less, by meticulous attention to technique.

Start the plan by simply jotting down every complication you can think of, each on a separate line and leaving a few lines between each. Then go through your list, making a note of one or two aspects of each complication: its importance, and by how much you will expand it in your full answer. Although the question asks about the *main* complications, it is best to start with a full list, later paying attention only to the main ones and omitting the obscure ones. If importance and expansion are rated on a scale of 0–4, then your list should look something like this.

Importance	Expansion	
4	4	Hypotension
3	1	'Massive' epidural
4	4	Dural tap
2	2	Unblocked segment, unilateral block
1	1	Retention of urine
3	1	Extradural haematoma
Last 3	1	Infection
1	1	Paraplegia
2	1	Paraesthesia
2	2	Motor blockade
1	0	Horner's syndrome
1	0	Puncture of fetal head, rectum (caudal)
4	2	Effects of drug overdose

A zero means you need no expansion at all; 1 means a single sentence is enough. Infection is an important complication because it is a disaster, not because it is common. Make a note to write about it in the final part of the answer.

Some might argue that motor blockade is not a true complication, but if a woman in labour does not like lying paralysed on her bed then for her it *is* a complication.

Add some notes to each complication.

Hypotension

physiology, fluids, vasopressors
aortocaval compression

'Massive' epidural

hypotension plus ventilatory support

Dural tap

immediate policy
later policy, analgesics, fluids
    blood patch (with details)

Unblocked segment, unilateral block

adjust catheter, position, dose; re-site

Retention

urinary catheter?

Extradural haematoma

clotting history, heparin, aspirin, pre-eclampsia

Infection

aseptic technique

Paraplegia

rare, role of adrenaline?, omit?

Paraesthesia

common, benign

Motor blockade

strength of solution

Horner's: omit

Puncture of fetal head, rectum: omit

Effects of overdose of drug/adrenaline:

suggested maximum dose

You should then group the complications for discussion. The first three, hypotension, the 'massive' epidural and the result of an unrecognized dural tap, for instance, fit quite logically in the same section. There is also the group of later complications.

There is a lot to write about and you must beware of trying to include too much in some parts of the answer, especially in your description of sterile technique and of the effects of overdose of local anaesthetic. Concentrate on the topics that score 4 in both columns of your list.

The question asks about *prevention and treatment*. When appropriate, it is better to discuss these two aspects together. Remember that prevention is much more important for some complications than for others; hypotension can be minimized by preloading with fluid and sensible attention to position and doses, whereas whether there are missed segments is largely a matter of luck. Just because the question asks 'Discuss the prevention and treatment . . .' does not mean that each aspect must be given equal weight in the answer.

1-8   What are the complications of spinal (subarachnoid) block?

OUTLINE PLAN

At the time

hypotension
  physiology
  dangers
  prevention and treatment
nausea
ventilatory insufficiency
failure of block

Postoperatively

headache
  cause
  treatment
urinary retention
others
  neurological
  infection/contamination

This question is similar to the previous one, but is less specific about the topic. The interpretation of the question is, however, the same: the examiners are asking for the causes, prevention, and treatment of the complications, not just for a list. Spinal anaesthesia has fewer complications than epidural anaesthesia, which is another way of saying that you will have time to give more detail. Because the effects on the cardiovascular system are likely to be more sudden and more pronounced than after an epidural block, hypotension is a good subject for an opening sentence.

> Some degree of hypotension is almost inevitable when a spinal anaesthetic is given.

But there is nothing wrong with a sentence that gives more of the overall structure of your answer rather than concentrating immediately on the most important complication.

> The complications that can accompany spinal block are divided into those that occur at the time of the block and those that occur later.

At the time

hypotension
  physiology
    peripheral
    adrenal
    cardiac
  dangers

> prevention and treatment
> posture, fluids, vagolytics, vasopressors

This is the main part of the answer, and you will have to give details of what treatment you would give for various degrees of hypotension. Subdivide hypotension into mild, moderate and severe; and write about young and old patients separately. Opinion is divided on when — and even if — vasopressors should be given. At Part 1 FCAnaes, an algorithmic approach will be sufficient; at Part 3, you should expect to be able to enter into debate about treatment with vasopressors.

> nausea
>   causes
>   action

It is not certain why patients feel nauseated, but the two important causes (because they can be life-threatening and can also be treated) are hypotension and hypoxia.

> ventilatory insufficiency
>   cause
>   treatment
> failure of block

Sedation often accompanies the reduction of afferent input, especially in the elderly. Partial obstruction of the airway secondary to this sedation is far more common than the ventilatory insufficiency of a high block. Phrenic paralysis is almost impossible after a correct lumbar spinal injection, unless the patient is tipped steeply head down, because of the small volume of injectate and the thoracic curvature. This is not true after a misplaced subarachnoid injection of the large volumes required for epidural anaesthesia, but you must take care in the examination that your thinking is clear. Note that the complications of spinal block do not include the complications of any drugs, such as sedatives, given at the same time.

Postoperatively
> headache
>   diagnosis
>   incidence
>   cause
>   treatment
> urinary retention

In the previous question, about epidurals, the treatment of spinal headache was more important than it is here, because persistent spinal headaches are unusual when the modern fine-bore needles are used. This question does not need the detail about blood patches required in the discussion of epidurals.

However, spinals are often the anaesthetic of choice in elderly men, in whom urinary retention can lead to prostatectomy at the same admission as the procedure for which they were admitted. It is this linking of general questions with real clinical practice that enables good candidates to impress examiners. Yes, spinals *can* be given to anyone, young or old; but in Britain they are more commonly used in the old, not least because there is a general dislike of regional techniques, but because the old are also more phlegmatic. You will not impress the examiners if you miss out an aspect of a topic because you have never seen it, but by all means emphasize those aspects that you are most likely to experience in your practice. They must be aspects directly relevant to the question. You may give all your spinals for transurethral prostatectomies, but TUR syndrome is not a complication of a spinal, nor does this question ask for advantages and disadvantages.

    others
      rare and unimportant
        labyrinthine disturbances
        cranial nerve palsies
      rare and important
        infection
        adhesive arachnoiditis
         transverse myelitis
         cauda equina syndrome
      common, but significance?
        backache

Much of this last part of the plan needs little expansion.

The question does not specify what drug has been given, but a 'block' implies anaesthesia, which can be obtained only with local anaesthetics; do not discuss opioids. There is no need to discuss overdose of the local anaesthetic.

1-9 Describe a technique for stellate ganglion block. What are the indications for and complications of this block?

OUTLINE PLAN

Location of ganglion

Chosen approach

    initial precautions
    patient position
    landmarks
    approach
    end-points

drug and dose

Result of blockade

Indications

therapeutic or diagnostic
in disease states
after trauma
to aid vascular surgery

Complications

injection into the vertebral artery
pneumothorax
perforation of the oesophagus (infection)
hoarse voice
phrenic paralysis
brachial plexus block
extradural or subarachnoid injection

This question is for Part 3.

The question specifies 'a technique'; you can explain why you have chosen the technique you describe, but *only describe one*. The best opening sentence is the obvious one.

> The stellate ganglion is a sympathetic ganglion formed by the fusion of the lowest of the three cervical ganglia and the first thoracic ganglion.

Location of ganglion

Chosen approach

why
initial precautions
patient position
landmarks
approach
end-points
drug and dose

Result of blockade

A diagram is not necessary for the simple anatomy of the stellate ganglion. A diagram to describe the approach will be confusing unless you are a good artist.

Indications

therapeutic or diagnostic
in disease states
after trauma
to aid vascular surgery

The main use for the block is in the pain clinic. You should know some of the diseases in which the block is helpful, and for how long it is likely to be effective.

Complications
injection into the vertebral artery
pneumothorax
perforation of the oesophagus (infection)
hoarse voice
phrenic paralysis
brachial plexus block
extradural or subarachnoid injection

For each complication you need to explain why it occurs, how to avoid or detect it, and your response to it. Beware of the systemic–local approach to complications; the amount of local anaesthetic will not be large enough to cause signs because of overdose (fitting occurs because of high, direct cerebral concentrations due to inadvertent injection into a vertebral artery).

The question does not ask for contraindications to stellate block, but under 'Chosen approach: initial precautions' you should have mentioned that you would check the patient's history.

CHAPTER 2

Questions based on physiology and pharmacology

2-1 What is meant by total available oxygen (oxygen flux)? How can it be measured in clinical practice? What factors affect it and what therapeutic measures may increase it?

OUTLINE PLAN

Equation

Oxygen consumption

> oxyhaemoglobin dissociation curve (diagram)
> increased metabolism

Cardiac output equation

Measurement

> cardiac output: thermodilution
> oxygen content: saturation, partial pressure
> (research methods)

Increase

> by cardiac output: preload, contractility
> by content: give blood
> inspired oxygen
> dissociation curve
> (dissolved oxygen)

The obvious way to start the answer is with a definition of oxygen flux:

> The total available oxygen is the product of the cardiac output and the arterial oxygen content, and under normal circumstances it is 1000 ml/minute in the adult.

The plan should start with the equation for oxygen content, after which there should be a comment on oxygen consumption.

> $(1.34 \times Hb \times saturation) + (0.003 \times PaO_2)$
> O_2 consumption (250 ml/min)
> > oxyhaemoglobin dissociation curve
> > exercise, other causes of increased metabolism

You should substitute figures for a normal adult male in the equation and calculate the oxygen content. (The form of the equation here assumes saturation is taken as the fractional value or the percentage, that is 0.98 or 98%, and the partial pressure is in mmHg.)

A brief discussion, and simple diagram, of the dissociation curve will help explain why much of the combined oxygen cannot be used (which means that the term 'available oxygen' is a misnomer). The diagram will also be useful later in the answer.

Define cardiac output: rate × stroke volume

Measurement

cardiac output: thermodilution
oxygen content: from saturation
    from partial pressure
    comments on research methods

In your plan, you can of course abbreviate to $CO = HR \times SV$, but do not write that in the full answer. CO is anyway not a good abbreviation because it can be confused with the accepted abbreviations for carbon dioxide or carbon monoxide.

Details of equipment are not necessary; comments on the accuracy and appropriateness of the measurements are. Remember that you cannot measure content from saturation, whether derived from pulse oximetry or from an arterial sample; you can only infer it. Partial pressure is one level of inference further back, because you first have to infer the saturation. There are devices for measuring saturation accurately, and there are methods for measuring content directly but these are not used in clinical practice. No more than one sentence, stating this quite clearly, should appear in your answer; no matter how much you may be able to write about the Lex–O_2–con or van Slyke's method, these methods are not clinically practical.

The last two parts of the question (factors affecting available oxygen, and therapeutic measures) are better tackled together rather than in separate sections, otherwise the answer will be repetitive. Work methodically through the definition and equation, mentioning inspired oxygen, ventilation, venous admixture and dead space.

Improve cardiac output: by preload

by contractility

Increase content: correct anaemia

increase inspired oxygen
shift dissociation curve
utilize dissolved oxygen

There are other ways of trying to improve the balance between oxygen supply and demand. They include paralysis and artificial ventilation, prevention of hyperthermia, the use of hypothermia, and vasodilators to improve peripheral perfusion. These will affect *oxygen consumption* but the question is not about consumption, it is about flux: the product of cardiac output and arterial oxygen content.

2-2 What are the adverse effects of intermittent positive pressure ventilation? How would you minimize them?

OUTLINE PLAN

Respiratory: ventilation/perfusion, dead space
    shunt
    FRC, atelectasis
   try: large volumes at slow rate, ± PEEP
    barotrauma
      sites
   try: care with pressure

Cardiovascular: (normocapnia)
    venous return
    pulmonary vascular resistance
   try: maintain intravascular volume, altered I:E ratio

Renal and endocrine
    decreased renal blood flow
      ADH and aldosterone
        sodium and water retention

Possible opening sentences:

> The important adverse effects of intermittent positive pressure ventilation (IPPV) are secondary to the increased intra-alveolar and intrathoracic pressures.

> There are respiratory, cardiovascular, renal, and endocrine effects of intermittent positive pressure ventilation (IPPV).

> IPPV has many effects on the physiology of the ventilated patient.

The first sentence draws attention immediately to what is clinically important; the second provides a summary and can give a structure for the rest of the answer. The third is poor: the abbreviation is not defined and the sentence is a restatement of the question.

It might be worth adding another sentence in the opening paragraph to enable you to restrict your answer to the *direct effects* of IPPV, and omit complications from the placement of endotracheal tubes and secondary infection, not direct adverse effects of IPPV. If the question was, 'What are the adverse effects of prolonged intermittent positive pressure ventilation?' then you would have to discuss these.

Respiratory: physiological
ventilation/perfusion mismatch
increased dead space
decreased FRC
progressive atelectasis
try: large tidal volumes, slow rate, PEEP
mechanical (barotrauma)
large airway
alveolar
try: avoiding high pressure, sudden pressure changes

The word *barotrauma* is a buzz-word that must appear in this answer, and it is an important topic that needs expansion.

Cardiovascular: (assume normocapnia)
reduced venous return
effect of age, hypovolaemia
interaction with lung compliance
secondary effect on intracranial pressure
increased pulmonary vascular resistance
try: maintain intravascular volume, altered I:E ratio

Renal and endocrine
decreased renal blood flow
increased antidiuretic hormone
increased aldosterone
sodium and water retention

Many of the effects of IPPV, particularly on the cardiovascular system, will be modified by the $PaCO_2$, but the possibly deleterious effects of hypocapnia and hypercapnia should not be discussed here. A statement should be made to the effect that it is assumed that the patient is maintained with a normal or slightly decreased $PaCO_2$.

The peak intrathoracic pressure can be reduced by new modes of ventilation such as high frequency oscillatory or jet ventilation. By all means put in a sentence to this effect, but detail about these methods is not needed.

2-3   Describe the endocrine and metabolic responses to major surgery and how anaesthesia influences them.

OUTLINE PLAN

Hormonal changes
beta endorphins, ACTH, growth hormone, ADH, catecholamines, cortisol, aldosterone, glucagon, insulin

Metabolic consequences:

hyperglycaemia, free fatty acids, negative nitrogen balance, salt and water retention, oxygen consumption, increased body temperature, immune suppression, blood clotting

The four phases

Initiation factors

Other factors

Modification: allay anxiety

regional analgesia, high dose opioids
general care

Although the question asks about 'endocrine and metabolic responses', they cannot be separated because one is largely the result of the other. There are two approaches to the plan, and you might like to combine them. The first is to make separate lists of all the endocrine and metabolic changes; the second is to work back from what you as a clinician see happening postoperatively to the patient. Your essay will be repetitive if you base it strictly on the two separate lists, but the lists are a way of getting your immediate thoughts down on paper quickly.

The obvious opening sentence is:

There are many endocrine and metabolic responses to surgery, and they can be modified to a greater or lesser extent by anaesthetic techniques.

This is a restatement of the question. An expansion is better:

Major surgery induces the 'stress response' in which there is a complex alteration of physiology involving the endocrine, metabolic, circulatory, and immunological systems.

Or you could alter the focus from the cause to the effect:

Amongst the many effects of the 'stress response' are salt and water retention and an increase in catabolism.

Both these sentences introduce early the buzz-phrase of 'stress response'. They are not very exciting, though, and if you want to gain the examiners' attention immediately you could start with:

Despite numerous research reports in which efforts have been made to prevent the so-called 'stress response', there is still no hard evidence that the endocrine and metabolic changes have any clear detrimental effect on outcome.

Anaesthetists taking Part 3 FCAnaes should be able to do more than regurgitate facts; they should have opinions. You may believe that the stress response does cause harm to surgical patients; quote your evidence and say so.

Here are the endocrine and metabolic lists, probably somewhat longer than the more usual answer plan:

Hormonal changes

beta endorphins increase release of anterior pituitary hormones
ACTH increases cortisol & aldosterone secretion
growth hormone causes hyperglycaemia, lipolysis, protein synthesis
ADH causes water retention
catecholamines cause cardiovascular changes, glycogenesis, lipolysis
cortisol increases gluconeogenesis & lipolysis, immunosuppression
aldosterone causes sodium & water retention
glucagon causes glycogenolysis, lipolysis
decrease of insulin causes hyperglycaemia

Metabolic consequences

hyperglycaemia due to increased glycogenolysis and gluconeogenesis
   and decreased peripheral glucose utilization
increased free fatty acids from enhanced lipolysis
negative nitrogen balance due to muscle protein loss
salt and water retention
increased oxygen consumption
increased body temperature
immune suppression
increased blood clotting

These should then be discussed under headings:

Phases: adrenergic/corticoid

corticoid withdrawal
anabolic
fat gain

Initiation: somatic and autonomic afferents

wound hormones

Other factors: pre-, intra- and postoperative

Modification by anaesthetic:

allay anxiety
regional analgesia +++
high dose opioids
general care
   nutritional
   avoid infection

Of these, only regional analgesia abolishes (most) parts of the stress response, and then only while the block lasts — hence the +++ against it in the list.

'Other factors' includes things like the state of the patient when they present for operation, undue hypovolaemia, sepsis, hypothermia.

2-4 Define physiological dead space. How may it be measured? What factors may vary it?

OUTLINE PLAN

Definition

physiological, anatomical, alveolar dead spaces
normal value

Methods of measurement

Fowler's
Bohr equation
assumptions
$V_D/V_T = (PaCO_2 - PE'CO_2)/PaCO_2$
technique

Factors affecting dead space

age
size
head position
tidal volume
drugs
apparatus
haemodynamic effects
pulmonary disease
anaesthesia

The answer must start with a straightforward definition.

The physiological dead space is that part of the tidal volume which does not take part in pulmonary gas exchange.

More than any other group of physiologists, respiratory physiologists have a well accepted set of abbreviations. Many of these have subscripts and superscripts, which makes them difficult to write clearly in handwriting. Throughout the relevant section of his standard textbook (*Applied Respiratory Physiology*, 3rd edn.(1987) Butterworths, London) Nunn writes out 'physiological dead space' and 'anatomical dead space' in full, and your answer will look better if you do the same. Abbreviations are better in equations, and when discussing V_D/V_T ratio and aspects of $\dot{V}/\dot{Q}$.

Of course, you are likely to use abbreviations in your plan, but we have spelled them out here.

physiological dead space =
   anatomical dead space (explain)
     + alveolar dead space (explain)
       ($\dot{V}/\dot{Q}$)
normal value (V_D/V_T ratio)

The question asks specifically about measurement of physiological dead space. In normal healthy humans, the physiological dead space cannot be measured as different from the anatomical dead space. Provided you write this, you can describe Fowler's method. Almost everyone describes Fowler's method with nitrogen as the marker gas, although almost nobody has a nitrogen analyser. Capnographs are now used.

Methods of measurement
> Fowler's: (nitrogen) carbon dioxide concentration
>> against expired volume after a breath of pure
>> oxygen (diagram)
> Bohr equation: assumptions
>> (derivation)
>> $V_D/V_T = (PaCO_2 - PE'CO_2)/PaCO_2$
>>> other forms
>> technique
>>> air sample, arterial blood sample
>>> measure apparatus dead space

The usual form of the Bohr equation includes the term for arterial partial pressure of carbon dioxide where originally there was the alveolar value. The arterial value will give the physiological dead space, and the alveolar value the anatomical dead space, but there can be problems with using alveolar partial pressure. This book is not the place for this discussion, and there will probably not be time for it in a written answer. It is nevertheless something that all trainee anaesthetists should read about, and it is better to know the assumptions and derivation of the equation than simply to be able to recall it.

Factors affecting dead space
> age
> size
> head position
> tidal volume
> drugs
> apparatus

Drugs such as catecholamines, anticholinergics, and those that release histamine do alter the dead space, though this is usually a small part of their overall effects on breathing. Apparatus may increase dead space (masks, mouthpieces and collecting apparatus) or decrease it (tracheal intubation).

> haemodynamic effects
>> posture
>> hypovolaemia and controlled hypotension
> pulmonary disease

anaesthesia
atelectasis
alteration of pulmonary vasomotor activity

Discussion of ventilation/perfusion ratio is relevant here, but there will not be time for great detail. At some point, it is worth mentioning the clinical relevance of dead space, such as the effect it has on capnography and in the design of paediatric breathing systems.

2-5   What are the adverse effects of oxygen therapy?

OUTLINE PLAN

Effects of oxygen itself

central nervous system toxicity
pulmonary

Effects secondary to physiological changes

respiratory
with blunted carbon dioxide response
absorption collapse
cardiovascular

Others

in neonates
anaemia
fire

Opening sentences:

Potentially lifesaving in many situations, oxygen should not be used indiscriminately because of a number of disadvantages, mostly related to the inspired concentration and the duration of exposure.

Oxygen has some adverse effects directly due to the oxygen and some due to secondary physiological changes.

These sentences are satisfactory but dull. Some interest is generated by:

The best known adverse effects of oxygen are retrolental fibroplasia in premature neonates and ventilatory depression in those with severe chronic obstructive airways disease, but far more patients have benefited from being given oxygen than harmed by excess of it.

The first half of this last sentence, up to the comma, is itself a reasonable start; the second half puts the topic into perspective.

Although it can sometimes be better to start with common things and work through to those less common, that approach is difficult to structure in this question. Start with the adverse effects of oxygen itself.

Effects of oxygen itself
   central nervous system toxicity
      mechanism, occurrence
      manifestations, treatment
   pulmonary
      mechanism, occurrence
         histology
      manifestations, treatment

There has been much study of pulmonary oxygen damage and for Part 3 FCAnaes you must have your own ideas of how important it is to consider the possible damaging effects of oxygen in patients who cannot be oxygenated unless they are given high inspired concentrations. This aspect of the question is less important, and warrants only a sentence or two, for Part 1.

Effects secondary to physiological changes
   respiratory
      with blunted carbon dioxide response
         (danger exaggerated)
      absorption collapse
      reduction of lung surfactant
   cardiovascular
      myocardial depression
      vasoconstriction

Every medical student knows that if you give oxygen to chronic bronchitics, they stop breathing. This is responsible for countless patients, from asthmatics to those who have just suffered cardiac arrest, being given 24% Ventimasks™. One of the qualities above many others that examiners seek, especially in clinical examinations, is a sense of proportion. So some discussion of the topic is needed, without exaggerating the dangers, and the sense of proportion will be expected at Part 1 just as much as at Part 3. The other topics need some expansion but, of these, only absorption collapse is controversial.

There are then a number of other unconnected effects.

Others
   in neonates
      retrolental fibroplasia
      (bronchopulmonary dysplasia)
   anaemia
   drug interactions
   physical
      fire

Bronchopulmonary dysplasia is in brackets because the main cause is probably secondary to barotrauma, which is not an effect of oxygen therapy. Increased risk of fire may not be a true 'adverse effect' of oxygen therapy, but it needs only a sentence to include it.

2-6 Discuss the desirable properties and the unwanted side-effects of nitrous oxide.

OUTLINE PLAN

Desirable properties
blood/gas solubility
   rapid uptake and recovery
   (concentration and second gas effects)
analgesic
   carrier gas of general anaesthesia
   decreases requirement of volatile agents
   Entonox
non-irritant, non-flammable
little ventilatory depression

Unwanted side-effects
hypoxia
pressure effects
awareness
circulatory depression
(support of combustion)
vitamin B_{12}

Some possible approaches to the opening sentences:

> The main advantages of nitrous oxide are that it is relatively insoluble and is a good analgesic, while the main disadvantages are its low potency and the danger of hypoxia.

> Nitrous oxide has been in use for 150 years and is still one of the most commonly administered anaesthetic gases.

> Nitrous oxide is supplied under pressure from cylinders or pipeline and is usually given at concentrations of 50–67% of the carrier gas mixture.

> Nitrous oxide was first prepared by Priestley in 1772 and its analgesic properties were first described by Davy in 1799.

The first sentence is the best. It tells the examiner that the candidate knows what is important. The second sentence is also good, because it introduces the idea that it is generally safe. The third sentence supplies background information, but does not have immediate impact. The fourth sentence would be an excellent way to start an answer to 'Write an essay about nitrous oxide' but has nothing to do with this question. If you write historical introductions (and they do make an answer read well) get the dates right, and spell the names correctly.

Desirable properties

> low blood/gas solubility (0.47 at 37°C)
> > rapid uptake and recovery
> > concentration and second gas effect
> analgesic
> > as carrier gas of general anaesthesia
> > decreases requirement for other anaesthetics
> > Entonox
> non-irritant to the airway
> non-flammable
> little ventilatory depression

The first two topics need to be expanded. You must show you really understand why low solubility leads to rapid uptake. Remember the concentration and second gas effects are more of theoretical than practical importance. Detail is required about analgesia. The last three topics can be dealt with quickly.

Unwanted side-effects

> hypoxia: high inspired nitrous oxide, diffusion hypoxia
> increased pressure in body spaces
> awareness
> some circulatory depression
> theoretical support of combustion
> interference with vitamin B_{12} metabolism

The first two are the important topics. Awareness and hypoxia are not really side-effects but are consequences of the low potency of nitrous oxide. It is probably worth knowing some of the detail of the effects on vitamin B_{12} metabolism, but it is very easy to fall into the trap of over-emphasizing them. Some candidates will see this question as being primarily about these effects, but it is not and they should not take up more than 10% of the answer, at most.

2-7   What are the mechanisms involved in anaphylactic and anaphylactoid reactions? How would you manage a patient showing signs of such a reaction?

OUTLINE PLAN

Anaphylactic reactions

> antibody–antigen and histamine

Type I: IgE and mast cells, atopy
Complement: IgG

Anaphylactoid reactions

histamine but no antibody–antigen
prior exposure not necessary
alternative path for complement

Some examples

Recognition: cardiorespiratory signs, skin and mucous membrane signs,
clotting

Differential diagnosis: includes simple asthma

Management

immediate: (help), oxygen, CPR, fluid, adrenaline, salbutamol, steroids,
?abandon surgery
then: take blood
later: yellow card (testing and counselling)

This is a very large topic. The question does not mention anaesthesia specifically, but it is reasonable to plan the second part of the question as if you are in the operating theatre and the patient is showing acute signs of a reaction. The immediate management would be the same with a reaction occurring to any other drug in any other site, but imagining you are in the operating theatre, actually dealing with the situation, is generally helpful when planning the answer to any question that asks for detail of practical clinical management.

A possible opening sentence would be something like:

Acute reactions to drugs are important because they kill, sometimes despite early recognition and treatment.

It might be better, though, to start straightaway with the mechanisms of anaphylaxis.

Anaphylactic reactions

antibody and antigen ⟶ histamine release
needs prior exposure/cross-sensitivity
type I: IgE and mast cells, atopy, family history
classical complement-mediated reaction
circulating IgG
second exposure activates all complement

Anaphylactoid reactions

histamine without antibody and antigen
prior exposure not necessary
alternative pathway for complement

The amount of detail about, for instance, particular components of the complement system, will depend on the wording of the question and the level of the examination. Not much biochemical detail will be demanded at Part 1. It is for Part 2 FCAnaes that most detail would be required, though it would then be asked in the MCQ paper or viva as there are currently no essay questions in Part 2. Candidates at Part 3 will be expected to have retained a good grasp of what they learned for Part 2.

The second part of the question is different. *Severe* reactions are most likely after intravenous injection; patients are in immediate and acute danger and any anaesthetist must be capable of managing them. The second part of the question needs an introductory sentence such as:

> For anaesthetists, the most likely and dangerous time for these reactions is at induction of anaesthesia, though they can occur at any time to any drug.

It would then be worth adding a *short* list of the drugs most likely to cause these reactions during the course of an anaesthetic. Alternatively you could add examples of particular drugs in the description of mechanisms. Remember that any reaction is rare. Give figures for incidences if you know them, but do not worry if you don't; what matters is that you know which are important.

Some drugs: thiopentone, suxamethonium, alcuronium, plasma
substitutes, antibiotics
Recognition: histamine (and other vasoactive substances)
⟶ cardiovascular collapse, bronchospasm, skin and mucous
membrane signs, clotting abnormalities

Do not just write this list out without qualification, implying to the examiner that you think all of these occur in all reactions. Any one, or any combination, and in any degree of severity, can occur.

Differentiate from: simple overdose, syncopal episode, asthma, aspiration
Management:
immediate: Call for help. 100% oxygen, CPR if necessary, fluid (colloid
best), adrenaline, nebulized salbutamol, steroids. Abandon elective
surgery.
then: contact laboratory, take blood
later: fill in yellow card, skin and blood testing, counselling

Think before you write your full answer from this plan: cardiopulmonary resuscitation 'if necessary' means *if cardiac output is insufficient* rather than the more usual diagnosis of a primary electrical event — the electrocardiogram may show normal complexes; and 'abandon elective surgery' may not be possible.

Note that the first item in management is to get help. This is obviously more important the less experienced you are, but when a patient is dying on the operating table an extra pair of hands is always helpful even if all they do is to phone the laboratory and squeeze fluid into the patient.

Note that this question does not ask about prevention of reactions or for details of what is done with the blood samples that you take.

It is worth repeating that this is a contentious subject, which means that experts in the field hold firm and opposing views. The important thing at Part 1 is that you should know how to treat a reaction quickly; at Part 3 you should know something of the arguments by keeping up to date with editorials, leading articles, and letters in the correspondence columns of the influential journals.

2-8 Describe the properties you would wish for in an ideal neuromuscular blocking agent. Illustrate how close or remote currently available drugs are from your ideal.

OUTLINE PLAN

1. Non-depolarizing
2. Rapid onset
3. Duration of action
4. Recovery and reversibility
5. Cardiovascular side-effects
6. Histamine
7. Cumulation
8. Physicochemical breakdown
9. Altered physiology

You should be able to list — without needing to think — the important properties of the ideal inhalational anaesthetic agent, intravenous anaesthetic agent, local anaesthetic, and neuromuscular blocking agent.

No ideal agents exist. The problem with neuromuscular blockers is that the ideal agent will have a rapid onset, which implies high dosage; and high dosage implies side-effects, prolonged action, or both. This paragraph so far would make a good start to the answer; a simpler opening is:

> Although there is not an 'ideal' neuromuscular blocking agent, atracurium is the closest to this that is available currently.

You may think vecuronium, or one of the drugs currently under study, is more close to the ideal. Of course, you will have to justify whichever drug you choose; and that is the idea of the question. You can pass the question just by listing the properties (if correct), but you will impress only if you show you can put together a logical argument from the properties of the available drugs.

1. Non-depolarizing
2. Rapid onset
3. A comment about duration of useful clinical action

Duration of action of the ideal drug is partly personal preference. For a long operation, some would prefer a long-acting drug, some would choose to give intermittent increments of a drug of intermediate duration, and others to use an infusion of a short-acting agent: none of these is necessarily 'correct' or 'ideal'.

4. Rapid recovery and easy reversibility
5. No cardiovascular side-effects
   ganglion block; vagolysis; sympathomimetic
6. No histamine release
7. Non-cumulative, and inactive metabolites
8. Metabolism by physicochemical not biological process
9. Unaffected by altered physiology

There are two ways of tackling the second part of the question. One is a table with columns for the drugs, rows for the properties, and the boxes filled with + and – symbols. This is a useful, even essential, exercise during your preparation for the examination, but is not a coherent way of answering the question, which asks you to 'illustrate'. It also has the disadvantage that you have to remember the whole table.

A better way is to comment on specific drugs where they are relevant: a comment about suxamethonium at (1); d-tubocurarine, pancuronium and atracurium at (5); alcuronium and vecuronium at (6); pancuronium, vecuronium and atracurium at (7); atracurium at (8); and so on.

The question refers to 'currently available drugs'. At the time of writing, doxacurium, pipecuronium and mivacurium are still undergoing trials, but a short paragraph mentioning these agents would be a good way of finishing the essay.

Two topics to beware of: priming, and laudanosine as a possible toxic metabolite of atracurium. They have, in retrospect, occupied an inordinate amount of space in the journals.

Neuromuscular blockade is a popular topic for editorials.

2-9 Compare the cardiovascular effects of the commonly used inhaled anaesthetics.

OUTLINE PLAN

Volatile agents:
   primary cardiac effects and mechanisms
      contractility
      rate
   consequences
      oxygen consumption and coronary blood flow

    reduced systemic resistance
    pulmonary vasculature & hypoxic vasoconstriction
       secondary effects
          cardiac output, blood pressure
    arrhythmogenesis

Practical considerations

    type of ventilation
    concurrent drugs

Nitrous oxide

    sympathetic stimulation
    depressant with poor myocardial function
    increases pulmonary vascular resistance

In the Introduction we wrote, '. . . you are being asked to organize your knowledge so that you present to the examiner an appropriate amount of detail' (see p. 4). This question is a good example of this principle. If the question were 'Compare and contrast halothane, enflurane and isoflurane', then the answer could only include a summary of what is required for the answer to the question as phrased above; there would not be time for anything more.

By contrast, 'What is the effect of isoflurane on the circulation?' would require further expansion.

> Anaesthetics affect the cardiovascular system (CVS) by effects on contractility, heart rate and arrhythmogenesis, coronary blood flow, and the peripheral vascular system.

This opening sentence gives a summary and a structure. It may be reasonable to indicate the abbreviation CVS if you think you will use it later in the essay, but beware of abbreviating everything: an essay full of CBF (which could be coronary, cerebral or colonic blood flow), RAP, PVS, HR, and so on takes little less time to write but is much less clear to read. You should be able to write enough on the subject without using abbreviations.

You should next define the 'commonly used inhaled anaesthetics' (it will probably be easier to deal with the potent agents separately from nitrous oxide) and state that the baseline comparison must be at normocapnia.

    primary cardiac effects
       reduced contractility: enfl > halo > iso
          mechanism
       rate: halo down, enfl & iso up
          mechanisms
    consequence: reduced oxygen consumption
       halo > enfl or iso
       (consider with:)

    coronary blood flow: all down
    reduced systemic resistance: iso > enfl > halo
      mechanism
    pulmonary vasculature & hypoxic vasoconstriction
    secondary effects: right atrial pressure, cardiac output, blood
      pressure
    arrhythmogenesis

Practical considerations

    spontaneous vs. artificial ventilation
    concurrent drugs

There is a lot of published work about the effects of these agents, but much of it is in animals. The actual effect of a specific agent in a specific patient will depend on such things as the autonomic balance at the time. All this, and topics such as the possibility of coronary steal with isoflurane, can be discussed under *practical considerations*. No-one has shown clear and important differences in outcome. Read around the subject and form your own opinions.

Nitrous oxide

    sympathetic stimulation
    depressant with poor myocardial function
    increases pulmonary vascular resistance

Ether, trichloroethylene, methoxyflurane and cyclopropane are not used commonly and discussion of them, no matter how correct, will gain you nothing.

2-10 Describe how you would evaluate a new inhalational anaesthetic agent for use in general anaesthesia.

OUTLINE PLAN:

Manufacturer's role

Volunteer studies:

    MAC, physiology

General form of clinical trials

    effect on MAC
    comparative studies
      physiology & anaesthesia
    specialized anaesthesia
    long-term (yellow card)

A specific question

    design (some detail)

> collecting data
> analysis

This is a difficult question. The process from the initial development to the licensing and then the clinical testing of a new drug is long and involved. Anaesthetists should be aware of what the manufacturer has to do before the drug can be used at all on humans, but most will play no part in the process until clinical trials. Except in the centres selected for the initial trials, most anaesthetists are likely to become involved in evaluation only in the later comparative studies.

Our approach to the question is to assume the agent has become generally available, summarize what the manufacturer will have done, and concentrate on a comparative study. This is easiest to do by outlining the sorts of question that could be asked, and giving an example of how to ask a specific question. You *could* go into more detail about more of the possible questions, but we suggest that you would find it difficult in the allotted time.

This is not a question about 'the ideal inhalational anaesthetic agent'; in some ways it is asking 'How would you conduct a clinical trial on an inhalational anaesthetic agent?'

Opening sentences:

> Before a new inhalational agent is introduced into clinical practice, the manufacturer will have investigated its physicochemical properties and completed animal studies. Initial dose-finding and descriptive studies will have been done in volunteers.

The only expansion you might need here is what happens in studies on volunteers.

Volunteer studies
> initial determination of MAC
> effects on physiology: immediate
>   late
> (toxicology)

Immediate physiology covers variables measured at the time; late physiology includes measures of hepatic function and haematological variables. There is no need for detail about toxicology but the word should appear somewhere.

The later clinical trials can concentrate on any aspect of the use of the agent. In this part of the answer you should mention the Committee on Safety of Medicines (known as the CSM).

General form of clinical trials
> effect of factors (e.g. age) on MAC
> comparative studies with another agent

general ease of use
induction
physiology
emergence
recovery
specialized anaesthesia
obstetrics
the pregnant woman
paediatrics
neurosurgery
cardiac surgery
long-term
unforeseen problems (yellow card)

In the last part of the answer, choose a question and outline a clinical trial to answer it. It is tempting in clinical trials to try and answer as many questions as possible, but better results often come from trying to control as much as possible while answering one simple question well.

Question
design
measured variables
avoiding bias
randomization
double blind
confounding factors
number of patients (exclusions)
pilot study
statistician
ethics committee
collecting data
analysis

Choosing illustrations to fit your question is better than trying to include everything. For example, if you have chosen to compare the incidence of nausea in the recovery ward for patients given either the new agent or isoflurane, a confounding factor would be drugs used for postoperative pain relief.

Do not mention using the agent for sedation or for the pain of labour; the question asks specifically about general anaesthesia.

2-11 Discuss the mechanism of action and use of spinal opioids.

OUTLINE PLAN

Receptors and pathways

Pharmacokinetics
intrathecal and epidural uptake and removal
Drugs, doses, methods
Indications
Side-effects
ventilatory depression:
others

This question is a general question about the action of opioids at the spinal level. There are many opioids in use clinically and there is no need to know in great detail about all of them. There is enormous scope for an infinite number of clinical trials using this or that opioid in ranges of dosage, with or without local anaesthesia, for a range of different operations. In reality, clinical anaesthetic practice would probably be little altered if the only available opioids were morphine, diamorphine, fentanyl and alfentanil — and some might argue that the last two are overused. Diamorphine and fentanyl are probably the opioids most commonly used by the perispinal route in Britain.

The examiners try to ask questions that are unambiguous. This question is not perfect. What is meant by 'spinal'? Does it include the epidural route? There will be an examiner in the examination room for at least part of the time during the examination, and you are free to ask them questions of interpretation. Otherwise, a useful tactic is to use the opening sentence to define how you interpret the question, for instance:

Opioids are given more commonly by the epidural route, but the mechanism of action is the same whether given this way or directly into the cerebrospinal fluid (CSF).

Other possible opening sentences:

The delivery of opioids directly at the level of the spinal cord gives better pain relief for a lesser dose of opioid.

Spinal opioids relieve pain by action on both spinal and supraspinal opioid receptors.

Not all anaesthetists believe in epidural opioids; some maintain that epidural opioids by catheter are a complicated way of giving a systemic infusion.

Receptors
mu1: analgesia spinal & supraspinal
delta: analgesia spinal & supraspinal
kappa: spinal
(mu2, sigma: not analgesia or not spinal)
Inhibitory spinal pathways
large afferent A-beta fibres (close gate)
descending inhibitory fibres (peri-aqueductal grey)

The discussion of which drugs to use is best incorporated into the discussion of pharmacokinetics, as fat solubility is so important to onset of action and likelihood of spread within the CSF.

Intrathecal
uptake:
    diffusion into spinal cord
    lipophilic drugs: rapid onset, e.g. fentanyl
    hydrophilic: slow onset, longer duration, greater incidence respiratory
        depression, e.g. morphine
removal
    diffuses back into blood supply of the cord, CSF, extradural space

Extradural
uptake:
    dural transfer, then as intrathecal
    systemic absorption
    (extradural fat)
removal
    epidural veins
    from sites of action: as intrathecal

The plan for epidural will be omitted if you have decided 'spinal' means strictly intrathecal.

For any drugs that you wish to discuss but have not mentioned yet:

Drugs (preservatives), **doses**, **methods** (single-shot, catheter)

As mentioned above, there is no need to list every drug that has ever been given. A *brief* comment about giving opioids and local anaesthetic drugs together would be sensible here.

Indications
    postoperative pain
    fractured ribs
    obstetrics
    terminal pain

The plan must then include the side-effects.

Side-effects
    ventilatory depression
        age, dose, route, water or lipid solubility; concurrent systemic opioid
    nausea and vomiting
    urinary retention
    itch
    neurological risk
        (arachnoiditis — safety of new drugs?)

We do not know if there will be long-term problems from injecting these substances perispinally. In general, older and more familiar drugs are safer — until proved otherwise — than newer drugs introduced with supposed but often very slight clinical advantages: arachnoiditis is a high price to pay for relief of postoperative pain. General comments of this sort, if appropriate, will make your answer interesting and help it stand out from the others.

CHAPTER 3

Physics, measurement and equipment

3-1 What are the safety features of the anaesthetic machine?

OUTLINE PLAN

Pipelines

Cylinders

Flowmeters

Vaporizers

Back-bar

Fresh gas outlet

Other

The anaesthetic machine is what was formerly called the Boyle's machine; it extends from the cylinders or pipeline to the fresh gas outlet. It does not include oxygen plants or the anaesthetic breathing system. The best opening sentence should define the machine to the examiner:

> The anaesthetic machine extends from the cylinders or pipeline to the gas outlet and there are safety features at the pipelines, the cylinders, the flowmeters, the vaporizers, the back-bar, and at the fresh gas outlet.

This gives a logical list, and examiners are always more impressed by an answer consisting of a logical sequence of facts than they are by an answer consisting of relevant facts not in a logical sequence.

Pipelines
    non-compressible
    non-interchangeable

Cylinders
    colour
    pin index
    reducing valve
    flow resistor

Flowmeters
    identification

hypoxic mixture protection
bobbin, static
top spring

Vaporizers

selection
filling

Back-bar

pressure-relief valve
oxygen failure

Fresh gas outlet

emergency oxygen

Other

anti-static
pipes and electric cables
modern machines

Many modern machines have integral monitoring and integral ventilators with in-built safety features. There are some machines with automatic record-keeping. A sentence about this is not out of place (mentioning delivered oxygen monitoring especially), but monitoring of the patient is not a safety feature of the machine that should be expanded in the answer to the question as worded, a question that perhaps will become obsolete as the newer more integrated anaesthetic machines become more common.

For Part 1, little more than writing out the list will be required. For Part 3, the candidate will have to give detail about the reducing valves, flowmeters, and oxygen failure devices. A common pitfall is mistaking the purpose of the pressure-relief valve on the back-bar: it is there to protect the machine, not the patient.

If you omitted the items listed under 'Other', then you might not fail the question, but you could not achieve a good pass at Part 3. If you forgot to mention the oxygen failure alarm, you would fail at both Parts 1 and 3.

The workings of the insides of vaporizers is not part of this question.

3-2 Give an account of the advantages and disadvantages of closed circuit anaesthesia with carbon dioxide absorption.

OUTLINE PLAN

Equipment

Advantages

economy, pollution, conservation

Disadvantages
efficiency, dust, resistance
knowledge and/or monitoring
    VOC (VIC)
complexity

Opening sentences:

The main advantage of closed circuit anaesthesia is that it is economical and the main disadvantage is that it is relatively complicated.

Closed circuit anaesthesia is used much more in the USA and Australia than in Britain, but the increasing use of new and expensive volatile agents may make it more popular in the future.

Closed circuit anaesthesia was popularized by Waters in the 1920s and is currently undergoing a revival of popularity in Britain.

There are two types of system for closed circuit anaesthesia, the to-and-fro system and the circle system.

In closed circuit anaesthesia, carbon dioxide is eliminated by absorption with soda-lime, which has advantages and disadvantages.

The first sentence is the best because it comes staight to the point. The second and third are good general introductions; the fourth allows immediate development of a first theme — a brief description of the equipment. The last sentence is weak.

Equipment
to-and-fro, circle (simple diagrams)
soda-lime

The diagrams of equipment need only be simple, but are useful later when discussing the dangers of misassembly of the circle.

Advantages
economy
less pollution
conservation of humidity and heat

Increasing use of isoflurane has encouraged the use of circles for economy; circles will be essential when new agents like desflurane become available.

Disadvantages
absorption not 100% efficient
inhalation of soda-lime dust
resistance
needs knowledge and/or monitoring

oxygen/denitrogenation
agent
VOC (VIC)
mechanically complex
malfunction, misassembly
cleaning

The two systems for closed circuit are very different, and it is in the disadvantage section that this can be discussed conveniently: some disadvantages are shared with the circle system and some are not. To anyone who has never used one, the to-and-fro system appears a convenient way of ventilating an intubated patient during transfer: it requires only a low flow of oxygen, and volatile anaesthetic vapour is retained in the circuit. Anyone who has used one will know that the canister is awkward to handle.

The complexity of circle systems is a disadvantage that needs discussion, which is why a simple diagram is helpful.

'VOC (VIC)' means *vaporizer outside or inside circuit*. With modern circle systems, the vaporizer is almost always VOC, which explains the brackets around VIC, meant to indicate that the answer should concentrate more on the problems of VOC.

Although the need for more monitoring is almost always quoted as a disadvantage, modern anaesthetic practice demands almost all the necessary monitoring anyway; monitoring of the volatile agent is now really the only addition.

3-3 Describe the features of vaporizers designed for use (a) outside (b) inside a circle breathing system.

OUTLINE PLAN

Efficiency

Resistance

Design

Delivered concentration and fresh gas flow

Features related to mode of use

An easy opening sentence is:

A vaporizer can be placed outside the circle (VOC) in the fresh gas supply or it can be placed inside the circle (VIC).

This gives no information to the examiner beyond defining the — here useful — abbreviations VOC and VIC. Your opening sentence should pick on one or two features of the two types of vaporizer.

Vaporizers designed for use outside the circuit (VOC) are of high efficiency and high resistance while those designed for use inside (VIC) are of low efficiency and low resistance.

VOC should precede VIC because it is the more common. You then need headings under which to discuss the two types. In the full answer, you could have a summary table immediately after the opening paragraph.

Efficiency

Resistance

Design

   type

   features

   examples

Delivered concentration

   related to fresh gas flow (FGF)

     behaviour at low flow

   related to setting

Spontaneous ventilation

Controlled ventilation

This is a short plan, but covers all the topics you need to discuss. Graphs can be helpful.

With some questions, especially the general clinical ones, the difficulty for candidates is (or should be) how to limit the answer to what is relevant in the short time available. This question is circumscribed and the danger for candidates is straying into irrelevance. No matter how much you know about closed circuit anaesthesia and how topical and important you think it is, the question does not ask about techniques. However, some aspects of technique can be discussed in a final section where they are relevant to:

Mode of use

   induction, maintenance

   advantages

   disadvantages

3-4 What features are desirable in an automatic lung ventilator suitable for use in an intensive care unit?

OUTLINE PLAN

The ventilator itself: use

   operation

   settings

   modes

PEEP etc.
backup
The ventilator itself: design
ease of use
safety
Other
humidification
nebulization
Cost

This is a big topic. The *adult* ICU is not specified, but we would suggest is implied unless the question asks specifically about paediatrics. If unsure, speak to the examiner in the examination room or write in your opening paragraph that this is your assumption.

Do not be distracted by the host of special features on modern ventilators, many of which are advertized by the manufacturers as if the intensive care unit is incapable of functioning without them. In-built metabolic computers, variable inspiratory patterns of flow, and a host of acronymic functions at the flick of a switch may make management easier for the staff, but they do not necessarily make it better for the patient. The most important single feature of a satisfactory ventilator for the intensive care unit is that it can cope with changing, sometimes rapidly changing, pulmonary mechanics. However, there are some patients whose mechanics are normal and stable, and they can be ventilated satisfactorily with inexpensive, unsophisticated equipment.

It is not an easy question for which to write a good opening sentence.

> Ventilators suitable for the intensive care unit (ICU) are almost universally constant flow-generators.

> Ventilators for the intensive care unit (ICU) need to be more versatile than ventilators in the operating theatre.

> One of the choices in selection of ventilator in the intensive care unit (ICU) is whether to use sophisticated machines with ancillary apparatus built-in, or relatively simple machines with separate ancillary apparatus.

Most discussions about ventilators start with the distinction between constant flow- and constant pressure-generators. That would be a reasonable start here (but do not discuss pressure-generators except to discount them), or it can be dealt with later when discussing pulmonary mechanics.

Use the appropriate abbreviation; if you choose to refer to the *intensive therapy unit* do not later write *ICU*. You should use the phrase chosen by the examiners, here *intensive care unit* and *ICU*.

The ventilator itself: use

  flow generator: volume preset
  tidal volume, rate, insp:exp ratio, (insp pause?)
  oxygen-air mixer
  ventilatory modes
  expiratory and inspiratory applied pressures
  monitoring and alarm facilities
  manual operation and emergency backup

Any number of variables can be monitored, with high and low set for each of them. You must discuss the problems as well as the benefits of alarms. An unqualified statement that 'The most sophisticated ventilators will be able to give alarms when the inspired oxygen, expired carbon dioxide, airway pressures, tidal or minute volumes are outside preset limits' is all very well, but the more possible alarms there are, the more actual alarms there will be, and the less useful each alarm becomes. A disconnection alarm (which may be triggered by volume or pressure) is essential, but many of the other changes will be noticed by the nursing staff before any harm could result.

When discussing modes of ventilation (such as IMV and MMV) and applied pressures (such as PEEP and CPAP), give the examiner your opinion of their utility. Like many other treatments that we use in difficult situations, these methods have their advocates and their detractors, and go in and out of fashion. The good candidate at Part 3 will know this; at Part 1, the emphasis will be on just knowing what is available for the uncomplicated ventilatory care of patients who do not require too specialized techniques.

The ventilator itself: design

  clear switches and dials
  size
  pipes and cables
  sterilization

Ventilator or ancillary

  humidification
  nebulization
  metabolic functions
  automatic recordings

Cost

It is less important to discuss topics in this second list than those in the first. A short discussion of costs is a good way of rounding off the essay. This is where you could comment on the choice between simple and complicated; it does not mean you have to know the price of half a dozen different ventilators.

3-5   Describe the physical principle of pulse oximetry and indicate its uses and limitations.

OUTLINE PLAN

Simple working description

Physics

light-emitting diodes (LEDs) and spectra

Output

information, display, alarms

Monitoring of saturation

human eye and cyanosis

examples

Monitoring of circulation

heart rate

blood supply

pulse wave form

Use in treatment

General limitations

Specific limitations

inherent

abnormalities

interference

dangers

An obvious opening sentence is:

Pulse oximetry is the most important advance in monitoring of the last few years.

This is harmless but is of little value if made without justification. A summary of function gets you straight into the meat of the first part of the question:

Pulse oximetry measures the arterial oxygen saturation non-invasively and accurately to within 1–2%.

Before describing the physics, the first paragraph can be completed with a simple description of the probe.

Probe

position

light-emitting diodes (LEDs), detector

Physics

absorption spectra

pulsed LEDs and ambient light

> two wavelengths
> pulsatile absorption (relation to other absorbance)

Output:

> pulse, saturation
> types of display, alarms

Pulse oximetry is obviously useful in many circumstances, and there is no need to give an exhaustive list. Better to choose one or two examples and explain why this monitor is especially useful. Do not forget to write down why it *is* so useful:

Saturation

> human eye and cyanosis
> examples of value

Another reason why you should not simply write 'The pulse oximeter is useful during routine and emergency anaesthesia, in the recovery ward, when opioids have been given peridurally . . .' is that there is *no need* for the monitor *all the time*. Tell the examiner when you think you should use pulse oximetry.

Circulation

> simple pulse monitor
> in vascular and microvascular surgery
> circulatory adequacy in contorted limb
> with cuff (for blood pressure)
> pulse wave form
>> arrhythmias
>> amplitude

In treatment

> adjusting PEEP
> deliberate hypoxia in premature neonate
> effectiveness of cardiopulmonary resuscitation (CPR)

All monitors have limitations, and this section should start with a broad statement about the anaesthetist being distracted from the patient, about believing the monitor when it is in conflict with clinical judgement, and the problems of alarms.

General limitations

Specific limitations

> inherent
>> not arterial oxygen tension
>> response time
>> low output, vasoconstriction, venous congestion
> abnormalities

>   of haemoglobin
>   pigments
>   on skin
>   in blood
>   pulses
>   external interference
>   diathermy
>   ambient light
>   motion artefact
>   dangers
>   trauma from probe

3-6   Discuss the indications for humidification of inspired gases. Evaluate the methods available.

OUTLINE PLAN

Basic physics

Clinical reasons

Indications

>   tracheostomy
>   tracheal intubation
>   respiratory tract infection
>   other

The ideal humidifier

Types

>   warm water bath
>   condenser
>   other simple devices
>   saline drip
>   cold water bottle
>   more complex devices
>   nebulizers

This is very much a 'bread-and-butter' question; it would be difficult to score highly on it, but similarly it ought to be a question that is difficult to fail. As the postgraduate anaesthetic examinations are pass/fail, that makes these questions — tedious though they can be — good questions to choose to answer if you have the choice. When discussing *methods* you should describe the physical principles.

Start with the normal physiology, which you can refer to in the opening sentence.

Inspired air is normally warmed and humidified in the upper airway.

Air is normally saturated with water vapour by the time it reaches the trachea.

Anaesthetic gases are dry, but this does not usually cause difficulties unless their use is prolonged and the upper airway is bypassed.

By all means give figures for relative and absolute humidity if you know them, but it is better to give no figure than confidently to give the wrong one. The first physical principle to mention is the relation between humidification and heat.

Physics: latent heat of evaporation

Clinical

> dry membranes, crusting, atelectasis
> inhibition of cilia

Indications

> tracheostomy
> tracheal intubation

Begin with the situation in which humidification is always used: patients on the intensive care unit, especially those with a tracheostomy. You can then discuss when you might discontinue humidification, and why it is less important in routine anaesthesia.

> respiratory tract infection (esp. upper)
>> children
>> adults
> other
>> drug delivery
>> rewarming in hypothermia

Your answer may become repetitive if you now write a list of methods, each with their advantages and disadvantages. A useful device is to give your requirements for the ideal humidifier.

Ideally

> tracheal gas to have satisfactory physical properties
> simple to use and service
> with any gases or mode of ventilation
>> any ventilator or system
> safe
>> temperature, hydration, electrical

That the humidifier can be used with any system implies that it does not affect the mechanical properties of the system significantly. This is especially important if the patient is breathing spontaneously through the device.

As with any list, the order in which you describe the devices should be logical. You can simply list them.

saline drip
condensers
cold water bottle
warm water bath
nebulizers

This is logical (in order of complexity) but suggests you are repeating a list from a textbook. The best plan is to *list* them in this way (because it is a logical way of *remembering* them) but describe them *as they are used commonly*.

We suggest that the order is:

warm water bath (with detail)
condenser (for operating theatre)
other simple devices
    saline drip (to dismiss)
    cold water bottle
more complex devices
    nebulizers

Nebulizers are described in the textbooks. At Part 3 you will be expected to know about them, but they are uncommon.

To flesh the re-ordered list out a little:

Hot water bath
mechanism
disadvantages
    condensation
    variable efficiency
    infection

Infection is a hazard with any humidifier, but this hazard is probably greatest with the warm water bath, so is appropriately discussed here. Obviously, if the thermostat failed there would be a risk of scalding, but that is perhaps not a true disadvantage of this method and will have been discussed earlier under *the ideal humidifier* and *safety*.

Condenser
principle
advantages
    convenience
disadvantages
    inefficient
    increased resistance and dead space (children)

The last disadvantage is not *especially* in children but *only* in children. Beware of regurgitating lists of theoretical advantages and disdvantages without thought.

Other simple devices
saline drip (to dismiss)
cold water bottle: brief description

More complex
nebulizers
microdroplets: mechanism
types
Bernoulli principle
mechanical
ultrasonic
advantages
constancy
disadvantages
cost and complexity
hazard: supersaturation

The notes for nebulizers probably exaggerate the stress you should put on them. Of most importance in your answer is that you understand the clinical principles of the need for humidification, and the workings and disadvantages of the humidifiers that you are familiar with. Writing in your answer (briefly) about incidents that have occurred in your clinical practice in which patients have been, or might have been, harmed by faulty or misused equipment shows the examiner that you are a clinical anaesthetist.

3-7 Outline the check procedure for anaesthetic machines.

There is no outline plan for this question, as the whole answer is an outline to the procedure. **This Answer plan as presented here MUST NOT BE USED as a check-list in the operating theatre. You MUST be able to reproduce a full check-list, whether you obtain the original from the Association of Anaesthetists or from the manufacturer of a specific anaesthetic machine.**

This seems an easy question, and at Part 1 it is. The Association has issued a check-list that is available as a plastic-covered sheet suitable for hanging on a corner of the anaesthetic machine. There is no alternative to learning its contents off by heart, and for this answer you have the opportunity to reproduce it.

But at Part 3, it becomes a much more difficult question. One could question the reality of asking someone to regurgitate a check procedure 'cold', without having the visual cues that we all use in practice when faced with a machine at the start of a list. There are all sorts of problems with using check-lists, and Part 3 candidates must be aware of them. Should there be a check-list to tick off? Must the check-list be witnessed?

What happens if there are two anaesthetists involved in a case, one after the other? How do you know someone has not tampered with your machine between cases while you have been in the recovery room? What if someone has refilled or refitted a vaporizer without informing you? What legal standing do check-lists have? Where should the check be recorded?

The use of check-lists is one of the most controversial topics in anaesthesia and candidates for Part 3 must have formed their own opinions that they are prepared to support when questioned by examiners.

There is no need for an opening sentence; you could just start with the start of the procedure. However, particularly at Part 3, it helps put some purpose into your answer.

> Check procedures should be performed at the beginning of each operating theatre session and are the responsibility of the anaesthetist.

> In all the surveys of critical incidents, lack of familiarity and failure to check equipment are important factors.

> Check procedures for anaesthetic machines are a good way of pre-empting many simple hazards, but the anaesthetist must realize that they do not ensure that equipment will not malfunction.

After that, the answer is a list, which comes under the headings:

Oxygen analyser

Medical gas supplies
disconnected and 'off'
cylinders and flowmeter control valves
primary audible alarm and oxygen failure protection device
pipelines
emergency oxygen

Vaporizers
fitting
flow
filling port

Back-bar
pressure relief valve

Breathing systems
inspect the configuration for leaks and obstructions
check expiratory valve
    specific problems

Ventilator
check normal operation
check pressure relief valve

    disconnection alarm
    availability of alternative means of ventilation
    specific problems

Suction equipment

The problem of small leaks

As examples of specific problems, you could discuss how to check the integrity of a Bain coaxial system, or how to check the unidirectional valves on the circle system.

We must repeat: Do not use the list as presented here as a check-list in the operating theatre. You MUST be able to reproduce a full check-list, whether you obtain the original from the Association or from the manufacturer of a specific anaesthetic machine.

CHAPTER 4

General anaesthesia

4-1 Describe the methods which can be used to monitor the depth of anaesthesia during surgery.

OUTLINE PLAN

Clinical signs

Isolated forearm

Electroencephalogram
  raw EEG
  cerebral function monitor
  computer analyses
  main problems

Evoked potentials

Oesophageal motility

(Frontalis muscle electromyogram)

Possible opening sentences:

> There is not yet any way of measuring depth of anaesthesia precisely, and clinical signs and experience are the best way of ensuring that patients are adequately anaesthetized and not aware.

> A reliable signal of anaesthetic depth would ensure that no patient was aware or given too much anaesthetic agent, and would also make it possible to have true feedback control of anaesthesia.

> Clinical signs of anaesthetic depth can be unreliable in patients who are paralysed and ventilated, which has led to the investigation of more sophisticated techniques.

> An important duty of the anaesthetist is to ensure that patients are unaware during operations.

> Many methods of monitoring anaesthetic depth have been described.

The first three sentences are better than the last two. The last sentence is the weakest; it is just a restatement of the question.

Candidates in vivas, when asked this question, sometimes offer the cerebral function monitor before clinical signs. This does not impress examiners.

Clinical signs: (Guedel) breathing, laryngospasm, swallowing, heart rate and blood pressure, pupils and lacrimation, sweating, movement
Isolated forearm: some circumstances

This section of the answer should make some reference to Guedel's signs. There is no need to reproduce them in any detail.

Practically, this is all most anaesthetists will use, together with a knowledge of the drugs. If awareness is the concern, then we know that 0.6 MAC of any of the modern volatile agents (although more for the first 10–15 minutes) in 67% nitrous oxide will keep virtually everybody asleep, and there are very few patients for whom this is not possible. None of the other techniques uses equipment that is routinely available. However, for Part 3 you will certainly be expected to know something about them.

Signals derived from electroencephalogram

raw EEG: brief physiology: basic waves, basic changes; too complex
cerebral function monitor: single bipolar lead, simple signal of amplitude and frequency; crude
computer analyses: spectral arrays and methods of representing changes in power and frequency.

There are many ways of dealing with electrical signals of neurological function to make them more easily interpretable by clinicians. Most methods depend on mathematical theory that clinicians cannot be expected to understand, but candidates for Part 3 should be familiar with terms like *spectral edge* and *median power frequency*.

main problems: requires expertise, depends on particular drugs and agents, expensive, operating theatre is electronically noisy
Evoked potentials: brief physiology: auditory, somatosensory, visual
even more experimental, problems as above
Oesophageal motility: spontaneous and provoked contractions. Poor specificity
Frontalis muscle electromyogram: experimental

4-2 How would you monitor neuromuscular blockade? What are the criteria available for assessing recovery from neuromuscular blockade?

OUTLINE PLAN

Stimulus
supramaximal
pattern
apparatus

Train-of-four count

Criteria

define clinical recovery
patient unresponsive
drugs, breathing, movements
train-of-four
patient responsive
sustained effort
train-of-four
late recovery

This is a straightforward, uncomplicated question. Start with a straightforward, uncomplicated sentence.

Neuromuscular blockade is monitored by measuring the response to a supramaximal stimulus delivered to a motor nerve.

In neuromuscular monitoring, a stimulus is applied to a motor nerve and the evoked response assessed visually, by touch, or by using apparatus to measure the force produced or the electrical activity in the muscle.

More general possible introductions are:

Although small increases in airway pressure may indicate that neuromuscular blockade is wearing off, there is no clinical observation that allows true monitoring.

Failure to realize that a patient is incompletely reversed from neuromuscular blockade is a potential cause of anaesthetic disaster.

This last sentence could be used to introduce the section of the answer devoted to the second part of the question.

The plan should start with a description of the stimulus because satisfactory monitoring depends on the delivery of a supramaximal stimulus that is not so large that it stimulates the muscle directly.

Stimulus

supramaximal
definition
assessment in practice
pattern
single twitch
train-of-four
double burst
post-tetanic count
apparatus
nerves and electrodes
measuring force

clinically, quantitatively
measuring electrical response

All these methods of stimulation need to be described, but the question asks 'How would *you* monitor . . .'. At this stage of the question you should declare what *your* practice is and why. For most anaesthetists this means a simple stimulator box and visual or manual assessment of the train-of-four, with occasional recourse to the post-tetanic count. There is not time in your answer for an erudite comparison of the train-of-four and double-burst stimulation; this is a question about clinical anaesthesia.

Train-of-four count
number/equivalent single twitch height/extent of
block/clinical significance

That has answered the first part of the question. Note that there is no need for any description of neuromuscular physiology or pharmacology. The second part of your answer must start with clinical assessment:

Criteria
define clinical recovery
patient unresponsive to command
review drug history
breathing
twitchy movements
train-of-four
patient responsive
sustained effort, e.g. head lift
train-of-four
late recovery

You need to define 'recovery'. In the usual clinical circumstances it means the ability to maintain ventilation and clear the airway, but more subtle tests of fine movements will show impairment of function for some time even after the use of shorter-acting agents. These tests do not need lengthy discussion, but a 'good pass' will be unlikely if you do not mention them.

The question does not ask about diagnosis and management of failure to recover from neuromuscular blockade.

4-3 Discuss the causes, effects and management of unplanned hypothermia during anaesthesia.

OUTLINE PLAN

Causes
radiation

evaporation
(intravenous fluids)

Patients and operations

Effects

cardiovascular
respiratory
central nervous system
liver
biochemical, endocrine, haemostatic
postoperative
shivering

Prevention

monitoring
maintenance of theatre and patient temperature

Management

slow rewarming
high inspired oxygen
ventilation?

An obvious pitfall is to include hypothermia as a planned technique; the question specifically excludes this.

The physiological mechanisms for conserving heat are affected by anaesthesia, and patients commonly have a temperature of less than 35°C at the end of even quite short operations.

More detail of the physiology of the control of temperature is probably not needed, but detail is required of the ways in which heat is lost.

Causes

radiation, (convection, conduction)
evaporation
intravenous fluids

Patients and operations

neonates, elderly

Get the emphasis correct. As anaesthetists, it is easy to start thinking about heat losses because of what we do to the patients — ventilate with dry gases and give cold fluids. The losses from these two factors are negligible compared with the main causes of heat loss: radiation, and evaporation from surfaces. Remember evaporation occurs through the skin, not just from uncovered bowel.

It is common to think that transfusion of cold blood is an important cause of hypothermia. A 70 kg (70 000 g) human at 37°C (310°K), contains (70 000 × 310 calories). One litre of blood at 4°C requires 1000 × 33 calories to raise it to body temperature, which is negligible compared with the body's heat store. In addition, blood is almost always warmed to some extent. Clear fluids, which are stored at room temperature, are even less of a problem.

There are other adverse effects of rapid transfusion of cold blood, such as the direct effect on the right ventricle, but that is not for discussion here.

Although the manufacturers of condenser humidifiers list conservation of heat as one of the advantages, the humidification of dry gases is a small factor compared with other heat losses during surgery.

The plan should then move to effects, and the question becomes quite difficult. It is probably best to work through the body systems, but the physiology of hypothermia is complex and the clinical importance of each of these complex changes is uncertain. Clinically important factors are that drug metabolism is likely to be slowed; consciousness is likely to be regained more slowly; and shivering increases oxygen consumption. Do not waste time on complicated discussions of matters of less practical importance, such as the relation between the partial pressures and solubilities of the blood gases.

Effects
> cardiovascular
>> bradycardia
>> decreased cardiac output
>> vasoconstriction
>> ECG changes
>> arrhythmias
> respiratory
>> oxyhaemoglobin curve shifts to left
>> gas solubilities increase

Ventricular fibrillation occurs below 28°C: the sort of fact candidates learn for examinations. In how many cases will *unplanned* hypothermia occur to this temperature? The answer is virtually never. Don't waste time telling the examiners of interesting facts that are irrelevant to the question.

Effects (cont)
> central nervous system
>> decreased cerebral blood flow
> liver
>> drugs, citrate
> biochemistry
> endocrine
>> stress
> blood clotting
> neuromuscular
> postoperative
>> shivering

Most of this list needs little expansion; stress what is clinically important.

The question asks about *management*, but should include *prevention*. It is surprising that prevention was not mentioned explicitly in the question.

Prevention
> monitoring
> theatre temperature
> warming blankets
> cover patient and exposed viscera
> (use warm fluids: irrigation, infusion)

Management
> slow rewarming
> high inspired oxygen
> chlorpromazine to prevent shivering
> consider elective postoperative ventilation

4-4 Discuss the causes and management of intraoperative hypertension.

OUTLINE PLAN

Preoperative

Intraoperative
> intubation

Maintenance
> light anaesthesia
> hypercapnia
> action: first check equipment

Specific operations
> aortic clamps
> phaeochromocytoma, carcinoid tumour

An excellent example of a question for which it is important for you to remember — and to let the examiner know — that common things occur commonly.

> The usual reason for intraoperative hypertension is that anaesthesia is too light for the level of stimulus, particularly in patients who have pre-existing hypertension.

> The plan can reasonably start with a brief summary of your policy of assessing the patient with preoperative hypertension, but do not spend too long on it: the question asks about *intraoperative* hypertension.

Preoperative

assessment, definitions
  causes of hypertension
  action

Intraoperative

intubation
  physiological response
  treatment
    when
    with what

There have been many studies of the haemodynamic response to laryngoscopy. There is little evidence that it matters. Our blood pressure varies widely during our everyday activities and people have heart attacks and strokes despite having normal blood pressure. Intravenous lignocaine is widely mentioned as a drug for attenuating the response; in examinations many candidates write about it in essays or talk about it in vivas. Yet some studies have failed to show that it has any effect at all.

This question would be fair at either Part 1 or Part 3; every anaesthetist is faced with unexpected hypertension during operations. At Part 3, the good candidates will have read widely enough to realize that many aspects of our practice are not based on any clear-cut evidence.

Maintenance

relatively light anaesthesia
    straining on endotracheal tube
    drugs given, e.g. adrenaline
    hypercapnia
  action: first check equipment
    drugs

Specific operations

aortic clamps
  physiology, treatment
phaeochromocytoma, carcinoid tumour
  elective
    effects, treatment
  emergency

Phaeochromocytomas and carcinoid tumours are rare but must be mentioned at Part 3. Acknowledge their rarity, and describe their management in some detail. At Part 1, you should know what signs lead to suspicion of the diagnosis, but not details of management: the mortality from undergoing laparotomy for unsuspected phaeochromocytoma is over 60%, and you should call for senior help.

4-5 Discuss the causes, effects and management of postoperative vomiting.

OUTLINE PLAN

Neurophysiology

Causes
   patient
   operation
   drugs
   techniques
   postoperative

Effects
   distressing
   airway
   risk to operative result
   electrolyte imbalance

Management
   prevention
   immediately postoperatively
   later
   anti-emetics

Possible opening sentences:

Vomiting may be caused by direct stimulation of the vomiting centre, or indirectly by afferent stimuli from the chemoreceptor trigger zone (CTZ), gastrointestinal tract, or vestibular nuclei.

The causes of postoperative vomiting are complex and in the current state of knowledge it is impossible to prevent it completely.

When patients are asked preoperatively if they have had a previous problem with anaesthesia, vomiting is a common answer.

Anaesthetists may worry about opioids causing ventilatory depression, but it is the discomfort and embarrassment of retching and vomiting that worry patients.

The first sentence gives a direct lead into the neurophysiology of vomiting. The others are more general but lend interest and show that you care about the patient. The second sentence would do equally well as a final sentence to round off your answer.

Neurophysiology
   vomiting centre
   CTZ
   afferent inputs

CTZ is a reasonable abbreviation, and it is likely you will use the expression a few times in your answer. You should not overburden your answer with abbreviations, so avoid VC (vomiting centre) and GIT (gastrointestinal tract).

Causes
    patient
        age, sex, psychology, idiosyncrasy
    operation
        site, duration
    drugs
        opioids
        anaesthetic agents
    techniques
        spinals etc.
            hypotension
    postoperative
        hypoxia, hypotension
        gastric dilatation, ileus
        early feeding
        movement

Opioids are potent emetics, but resist the temptation to leap into this part of the answer with 'Morphine and other opioids commonly cause vomiting'. Be organized: patient, operation, anaesthetic, postoperative factors.

Effects
    distressing
    airway
        laryngeal spasm, aspiration
    risk to operative result
        bleeding
        eyes, neurosurgery
        jaw wiring
    electrolyte imbalance

It is worth mentioning jaw wiring specifically. Electrolyte disturbances occur only if vomiting is prolonged.

When it comes to management, deal with immediate and later postoperative vomiting separately:

Management
    prevention
    immediately postoperatively
        turn, clear pharynx
    later

> treat any direct cause
> reassurance
> anti-emetics
>> site of action, efficacy
>> side-effects

Prevention covers the avoidance of emetic drugs and the psychological approach to the patient. This occurs again as 'reassurance'. Nurses don't (or shouldn't) just shove a kidney dish under the patient's nose; they suggest the patient takes a deep breath, or breathes oxygen. Unless the nausea is caused by hypoxia, this is unlikely to have anything other than a placebo effect, which, for nausea, can be powerful.

If the essay asked 'Discuss the use of anti-emetics in clinical anaesthesia', you would have to include detail of all the classes of drug. In this answer, which has to cover far more than just the anti-emetics, by all means give a summary of the available drugs but concentrate on the ones that you use.

4-6   Outline the causes, effects and management of perioperative changes of serum potassium concentrations.

OUTLINE PLAN

Physiology

Summary of disorders

> common examples

Hypokalaemia

> causes
> effects
>> function of muscles
>>> cardiac muscle (emphasize)
>> metabolic changes
> management

Hyperkalaemia

> cardiac effects
> causes
>> excessive intake
>> poor excretion
>> shift from intracellular compartment
> diagnosis
> treatment
>> urgent
>> non-urgent

This is a difficult question. Except during complex procedures such as cardiopulmonary bypass or liver transplantation, the concentration of potassium in the serum is not measured during operation but is inferred from clinical knowledge or indirect information such as electrocardiographic changes. However, anaesthetists often need to know the serum potassium concentration before operation, for example in patients with renal failure or in unstable diabetics receiving an infusion of insulin. Present a cogent account of how to deal with preoperative abnormalities. Intraoperative problems are circumscribed and can be dealt with fairly simply. Postoperative abnormalities are really the same as preoperative, but without the temporal constraint of getting a patient fit for operation.

The answer will have to begin with a summary of the normal physiology of potassium, but the opening sentence is a good place to state the importance of potassium to anaesthetists, and when they are most likely to be concerned with it.

> Patients are at risk of fatal cardiac arrhythmias if the serum potassium concentration is too high or too low, either of which may occur in a number of common situations when patients present for operation, often as emergencies.

Other opening sentences are possible, but some approaches do not tell the examiner immediately that you understand why the question was asked.

> Potassium is the most important intracellular cation, its control is linked to that of sodium and acid-base balance and controlled by aldosterone.

> The normal serum potassium concentration is 3.5–5.0 mmol/L, and abnormal values for this mainly intracellular ion are more dangerous if they occur acutely.

Both these statements are true, but they fail to stress what is important.
Do not use K^+ as an abbreviation for potassium.

Physiology
    normal values
    control (brief)
    related physiology (sodium, acid–base)

Summary of disorders
    hypokalaemia and hyperkalaemia
      acute more important than chronic
     common examples
    principles of timing of operation

Hypokalaemia
    causes

After the opening physiology, have a paragraph that gives the important diagnoses that cause changes in potassium concentrations. At this stage of the answer this is not intended as an exhaustive list but, like the opening sentence, is intended to show the examiner that you can think sensibly. Too little — hypokalaemia — should logically be dealt with before too much.

> causes
>> decreased intake
>> increased loss
>> shift to intracellular compartment
>> others

Clinical examples are needed for all these headings. Choose common ones, and give the sort of reduction in serum potassium concentration that you would expect to measure. Do not just write 'Diuretic therapy can cause major reductions in serum potassium'. This is true, but which diuretic; and what do you mean by 'major'?

An intraoperative cause worth mentioning here is hyperventilation.

The note 'others' includes oddities such as familial periodic paralysis, endogenous endocrine disturbances (infusions of insulin are common enough to come under 'shifts'), and the particular clinical situation of cardiopulmonary bypass. These are details for the Part 3 candidate.

> effects
>> function of muscles
>>> electrophysiology
>> clinical result
>>> smooth muscle
>>> skeletal muscle
>>> cardiac muscle (emphasize)
>> metabolic changes

The effects on cardiac muscle are the most important to anaesthetists.

> management
>> diagnosis
>> treatment: scheme, monitoring
>>> when ready for surgery?

Although the question asks about serum potassium, it is worth adding a comment that the serum potassium concentration can be normal even if there is marked intracellular depletion. You need to give figures for replacement: how much and how quickly.

The scheme for hyperkalaemia follows a similar pattern to that for hypokalaemia, except that 'effect' can be dealt with quickly at the beginning because the only one that matters is the effect on the heart.

Hyperkalaemia
> cardiac effects

> causes
> > excessive intake (especially stored blood)
> > poor excretion

'Poor excretion' obviously includes renal failure, but do not forget potassium-sparing diuretics, and for completeness adrenal insufficiency. A candidate at Part 1 would be expected to know the first two; a candidate at Part 3 ought to know of adrenal insufficiency.

> shift from intracellular compartment
> > suxamethonium
> > muscle injury and other conditions
> > metabolic acidosis (malignant hyperthermia)
> artefact (haemolysed sample)

This is an important section of the answer, which is more about intraoperative changes. Underventilation is an important cause. You will need to give details of, for example, the period of danger after burns. Malignant hyperthermia is given as an extreme form of metabolic acidosis. It must be mentioned, but there is no need for detailed description of the syndrome.

> diagnosis
> > ECG changes
> treatment
> > urgent
> > > calcium gluconate
> > > glucose and insulin
> > > bicarbonate
> > > when ready for operation?
> > non-urgent
> > > calcium resonium
> > > dialysis

Details of doses and monitoring will be needed.

4-7 What factors should lead you to anticipate difficulty with tracheal intubation? Describe the management of anticipated and unanticipated difficult intubation.

OUTLINE PLAN

Appearance
> mouth, teeth, throat, jaw, neck

Radiological signs:

Acquired conditions
> syndromes

Management (anticipated)

    intubated before?
    intubation necessary?
    no relaxant
    range of equipment
    awake intubation
    inhalational induction
    blind nasal
    cricothyroidotomy/tracheostomy
    intubating fibreoptic laryngoscope

Management (unanticipated)

    mask and airway?
        yes: continue (cricoid pressure if emergency)
            re-establish spontaneous breathing
        no: urgent establishment of airway
    consider postponing operation
    write clear notes, tell patient

An obvious opening sentence is:

> Failure to intubate is a major cause of morbidity and mortality associated with anaesthesia.

No examiner could argue with this, but it is a very bland and trite statement. An opening sentence should take the examiner's attention:

> Failure to intubate remains an important cause of death related to anaesthesia, and every anaesthetist must have a clear plan of what to do, especially for when difficulties arise unexpectedly.

Remember at some point early in your answer to write that it is not actually failure to intubate, but failure to ventilate, that kills people.

The plan should start with appearance of the otherwise normal patient — what you would be looking out for during the preoperative assessment. This could be presented as a list within the essay.

Appearance

    short muscular neck with full set of teeth
    protruding upper incisors and/or maxilla
    receding mandible
    poor mouth opening
    long high arched palate
    fauces and uvula not visible
    high larynx

Radiological signs

    increased alveolar–mental distance
    increased posterior depth of the mandible
    decreased atlanto-occipital distance

In practice, X-rays are unlikely to be available unless the patient is due for surgery to the head and neck, and few anaesthetists ask specifically for these films but trust their clinical judgement in anticipating a difficult intubation.

The plan should now move to the patient with acquired problems, arranged anatomically.

Acquired conditions
> restricted mouth opening
> restricted neck movement
> soft tissue swelling
> laryngeal
> tracheal

For each of these, an example or two should be given. Examples should be of common conditions — fractured jaw, ankylosing spondylitis, goitre, epiglottitis, tracheal stenosis (not common in itself, but post-intubation stenosis is probably the commonest cause of difficulties with intubation originating in the trachea) — and there is no need for exhaustive lists.

It is worth making brief mention of some specific conditions such as gross obesity, acromegaly, cleft palate and Pierre Robin syndrome, but there is not time in this answer to describe any of them.

Management starts with examination of the patient, but there is no need to describe this in detail as it is covered in the first half of the question. Faced with a patient who looks difficult, anaesthetists usually check the notes to find out if intubation has been successful in the past; this is the point at which to start the next part of the question.

Management (anticipated difficulty)
> intubated before?
>> change since last time?
> consider:
>> surgery with local anaesthesia
>> need for intubation
> no relaxant
> equipment: blades, tubes, bougies, laryngeal mask
> awake intubation
> inhalational induction
> blind nasal
> retrograde catheter
> cricothyroidotomy/tracheostomy
> fibreoptic: awake/anaesthetized

Specific management depends on the specific patient but this is a general essay. You will need to give an outline of each technique you mention. Some are choices (awake intubation or inhalational induction); some are progressions (inhalational induction, blind nasal, cricothyroidotomy, tracheostomy). If you suggest the progression from attempted blind nasal intubation to fibreoptic intubation of an anaesthetized patient, you are letting the examiner know either that you have never used an intubating fibreoptic bronchoscope or that you are an expert — the trauma from the blind attempts would make use of the fibrescope difficult.

The unanticipated difficult intubation allows you also to consider the special difficulties of the emergency operation. The assumption for unanticipated difficulty is that the patient has already been given a relaxant.

Management (unanticipated difficulty)
    can you ventilate with mask and airway?
        yes: as above (cricoid pressure if emergency)
            re-establish spontaneous breathing
        no: get help
            cricothyroidotomy
    consider postponing operation
        ?elective tracheostomy
    write clear notes, tell patient

Every anaesthetist must have a plan for managing the unexpectedly difficult airway, but it is no failing — even for consultants — to call for an extra pair of hands. Nothing is lost if the problem is solved by the time help arrives. Pride has no place in medicine.

4-8 What are the causes of unexpected delay in the return of consciousness after general anaesthesia? Describe your management.

OUTLINE PLAN

Prolonged action of anaesthetic drug

Altered physiology

Pathophysiology

Primary management
    breathing?
    review the anaesthetic
        investigations and treatment
    review the patient
        ?diabetic
        drugs, diseases
        investigations and treatment

Secondary management
    neurology
    recovery or ITU?

This is a standard question of everyday clinical management. It is difficult to know how the answers at Parts 1 and 3 might differ. Perhaps the candidate at Part 3 is expected to know more of, and more about, rarities — but therein lies a danger: at all levels of medicine, from clinical student onward, it is all too easy to get side-tracked by rare conditions.

The best way to answer this question is to imagine that you are in the operating theatre. The patient has been lifted off the table and on to the trolley, and you are beginning to worry because the patient is not waking up. Your thoughts at that moment should form the answer to this question.

Your first sentence should not be:

> There are many causes for the delayed return of consciousness after a general anaesthetic.

This is a prime example of the 're-statement' type of opening sentence, and it is a waste of effort: the examiners would be unlikely to ask the question if there were not a number of possible causes.

One possibility is to start with a sentence that lists the general causes, but probably best is to write:

> The most common cause of unexpected delay in the return of consciousness is an absolute or relative overdose of drug.

There is a large inter-patient variability of response to any drug, and most patients who fail to wake up when expected are those who are at one end of the range of response.

Lists can be drawn up:

Prolonged action of anaesthetic drug

>   volatiles, adjuncts
> absolute overdose
> increased sensitivity, e.g. age
> delayed elimination
> long-acting drugs

Decreased hepatic metabolism and decreased protein binding could theoretically have an effect, but no-one has shown any consistent general effect, and you should beware of detailed descriptions of how these processes *could* prolong wakening; the fact is they don't. The use of opioids in incipient hepatic encephalopathy is a different problem and can be discussed later.

Altered physiology

>   hypo- or hypercapnia
> hypoglycaemia
> hyperosmolar non-ketosis
> TUR syndrome
> hypothermia

Pathophysiology
  liver disease
  porphyria
  endocrine
    hypothyroidism
  cerebral events

Again, some of these are common; some are less common; and some are exceedingly rare. Your management should move from the obvious to the less obvious because that is what you would (or should) do. Your management should also stress the reversible. If you think of hypoglycaemia early, intravenous 50% dextrose may prevent cerebral injury, whereas not realizing in the first few minutes that the patient has had an unsuspected cerebrovascular accident is unlikely to do any harm.

Primary management:
  is the patient breathing?
    review the anaesthetic
    drugs and fluids
    ventilation
    circulation
    surgical events
  investigations and treatment as indicated
  the patient
    ?diabetic
    drugs, diseases
  investigations and treatment as indicated

This list for management can be discussed by referring to the lists of causes for specific investigations and treatment. You are now left with the rarer, most likely neurological, causes.

Secondary management
  simple neurological assessment
  observe in recovery or ITU?
  (contact neurologist)

The likeliest non-neurosurgical operation after which this problem may arise is carotid endarterectomy.

Left with a postoperative conundrum, you need to seek help. The question is 'Describe your management', and your management in practice would be to contact a neurologist. It would not be the anaesthetist's job to order a CT scan, so it should not be in this answer.

4-9   How does posture affect the anaesthetized patient?

OUTLINE PLAN

Physiological changes awake to anaesthetized

Cardiovascular consequences

Respiratory consequences

Anatomical considerations

Specific positions

The obvious way to answer this question is to work through the positions, discussing each one before moving to the next. This is bound to be repetitive, because almost all the effects of posture can be summarized under three headings: changes in respiratory function, changes in circulatory function, and considerations of anatomy. The most efficient answer discusses these in a general way, illustrating problems by referring to the positions that give most trouble.

The opening sentence could list the headings mentioned above, or could be a more general statement such as:

> Patients are usually positioned on the operating table for the surgeon's convenience, and the anaesthetist must realize the implications and minimize any ill-effects.

This next sentence is true but not illuminating:

> Different positions have different effects on the anaesthetized patient.

To round off the opening paragraph, list the usual positions.

> Patients may be placed supine, head-down, head-up, in lithotomy, lateral, prone or sitting.

Writing head-down and head-up is better than Trendelenburg and reverse Trendelenburg.

The plan then follows the general one of physiology — altered physiology — pathology in appropriate sections.

Changes awake to anaesthetized

loss of cardiovascular reflexes
primary effects
secondary respiratory effects
loss of ventilatory drive
to carbon dioxide
to added load
loss of muscle tone

Cardiovascular consequences

hypotension, pooling
elderly, diseases, drugs
compression of vena cava and aorta
cerebral blood flow

Respiratory consequences

FRC and ventilation/perfusion
   diaphragmatic splinting
   differential blood/air flow
cardiovascular interactions

Anatomical considerations

eyes, nerves, joints, limbs
access to airway and cannulae

Specific positions

lithotomy
prone knee–elbow
lateral
sitting

Throughout the essay, refer to specific positions as examples where relevant. It is not necessary to comment about every aspect of every position. The last section will allow you to comment on particular problems — such as air embolus in the sitting position — and perhaps to finish by discussing one difficult position, the prone knee–elbow position for instance, in detail.

4-10 Discuss the causes, diagnosis and treatment of oliguria occurring during the first 24 hours following laparotomy in a previously healthy patient.

OUTLINE PLAN

Prerenal

hypovolaemia
hypotension

Renal

prerenal progression
bugs, blood, dyes, drugs

Postrenal

ureter, bladder

Management

catheter
treat prerenal or postrenal causes

If renal

maintain renal blood flow
treat biochemical consequences
make specific diagnosis

investigations

treatment: short-term (long-term)

The important words in this question are 'previously healthy'. This implies that renal function was normal before surgery and there is no need to comment at all about preoperative assessment of renal function. The other important point of wording is 'oliguria' (i.e. not 'renal failure'). The commonest cause of oliguria after an operation is hypovolaemia, and that is a good place to start.

> The commonest cause for oliguria in the postoperative period is hypovolaemia, although there are other causes that should be considered.

Another possible opening sentence is one of definition.

> Oliguria is a urine output of less than 0.5 ml/min, or 0.5 ml/kg/hr, and it may be secondary to prerenal, renal or postrenal causes.

This gives a structure to the initial plan:

Prerenal: due to reduced renal perfusion

hypovolaemia

    intravascular fluid volume

    extracellular fluid volume

hypotension

    induced

    pump failure

Renal: due to ischaemia or nephrotoxins

unrelieved prerenal oliguria

    atheromatous embolization of renal vessels

septicaemia

incompatible blood transfusion

radiological contrast media

nephrotoxic drugs

Again, the commonest cause of established renal failure after surgery is hypovolaemia and failure to correct it. Atheromatous embolization is likely only after surgery of the abdominal aorta, but a patient with an aneurysm (less so with occlusive vascular disease) can be previously healthy. Most people think of aminoglycosides when considering nephrotoxic drugs, but intraoperative antibiotics given to a previously healthy patient will not cause oliguria within 24 hours. The non-steroidal anti-inflammatory drugs (NSAIDs) can cause renal failure, especially in the elderly.

You may be tempted to include conditions like hepatorenal syndrome, crush syndrome, and acute-on-chronic renal failure. With the possible exception of acute pancreatitis, which may be triggered by surgical manipulation, these are irrelevant when considering a previously healthy patient.

Postrenal: due to lower tract obstruction

ureter — pelvic surgery

bladder — blocked catheter

Management

catheter if in any doubt

treat prerenal causes

fluids, mannitol, CVP, dopamine

treat postrenal causes

The drug given most commonly to oliguric patients postoperatively is frusemide. Many believe that frusemide has no place in prerenal failure: it confuses the biochemistry, worsens hypovolaemia, and does not prevent incipient renal failure anyway. All it does is to confirm that the kidneys can or cannot pass urine, but there are other and better ways of reaching the correct diagnosis.

If renal

principles of management

maintain renal blood flow

treat biochemical consequences

make specific diagnosis

investigations

urine: SG, sodium, osmolality

blood: urine/plasma ratios

treatment

fluid restriction

potassium balance

acidosis

The question could be rounded off with a *brief* summary of the overall treatment for established renal failure. As the question asks you to consider oliguria *during the first 24 hours*, detailed discussion of nutrition and dialysis are irrelevant.

4-11 Give a critical account of prophylactic measures designed to reduce the incidence and consequences of pulmonary aspiration.

OUTLINE PLAN

Definitions

types of aspiration

Mendelson's syndrome

Increased risk of regurgitation

anatomy
obstetrics
emergency surgery
neurological
    altered conscious level
    impaired reflexes

If high-risk

drugs: antacids, H_2 antagonists, gastric motility

If at-risk

mechanical measures
    posture, rapid sequence induction
precautions at extubation

A *critical* account invites your own opinions. Describe your clinical practice: if you give metoclopramide to all your patients preoperatively, tell the examiner and say why. Writing 'this can be done and that may be done' is not a critical account.

The question asks for *prophylactic* measures to reduce the *incidence* and *consequences* of aspiration. Prophylaxis to reduce the incidence is easy: cricoid pressure is an obvious example. Prophylaxis against the consequences is more difficult to define: what about steroids and bronchial lavage? Are they *treatment* of aspiration, or prophylaxis against the consequences of aspiration? Use the opening sentence to define the scope of your answer.

> Prophylaxis against pulmonary aspiration means reducing the volume and acidity of the gastric contents, reducing the likelihood of vomiting and regurgitation, and reducing the likelihood of regurgitation becoming aspiration.

This is the interpretation we put on the question: that prophylaxis is what happens before aspiration.

Do not use *reflux* and *regurgitation* interchangeably: reflux implies gastric contents in the oesophagus; regurgitation implies gastric contents in the pharynx. Much of the work on which prophylactic measures are based was from measures of reflux. This is a good critical point worth mentioning somewhere in the essay.

Beware of this opening sentence:

> Mendelson's syndrome is the term used to describe the severe asthma-like reaction from the chemical pneumonitis caused by aspiration of a large volume of gastric liquid of pH less than 2.5.

This is true, but the question asks about pulmonary aspiration not Mendelson's syndrome. Of course, Mendelson's syndrome is important, but if you launch straight into it there is the risk you will forget about the dangers of aspirating beer and chips.

A better alternative, which also introduces Mendelson's syndrome early, is:

Aspiration of gastric contents is almost always a preventable accident, which in its most serious form, Mendelson's syndrome, causes a severe chemical pneumonitis.

The plan:

Definitions
> types of aspiration
>> vomiting and regurgitation
>> Mendelson's: definition, incidence, mortality

Increased risk of regurgitation
> anatomical: normal anatomy, hiatus hernia
>> obstetrics
>> emergency surgery
>>> bowel obstruction
>> raised intra-abdominal pressure
>> ?nasogastric tube

The latter is a good subject for critical appraisal: should you remove a tube before induction of anaesthesia?

> neurological
>> altered conscious level
>> impaired cough and gag reflexes
>>> recent extubation
>>> seriously ill patients
>>> bulbar palsy
>>> elderly patients

If high-risk:
> antacids
>> magnesium trisilicate, sodium citrate
> histamine-2 antagonists
>> action
>> cimetidine, ranitidine
> others
>> omeprazole
> gastric motility
>> metoclopramide

Brief mention of modes of action, doses, advantages and disadvantages are needed for all drugs.

If at-risk
> mechanical measures

posture: any unconscious patient
rapid sequence induction: full description
consider: awake intubation
extubation
conscious level
facilities in recovery room

We have not included any measures taken after aspiration has occurred. You may ask the examiner in the hall if the question does indeed include these aspects, but otherwise try this final sentence to show you realize that the examiner may have a different interpretation:

If, despite all these precautions, aspiration does occur, some believe that steroids, antibiotics, and bronchial lavage are helpful.

This is not a *critical* sentence (see above). You will need to give more details and reasoning if you think the answer should include these measures.

4-12 What precautions should the anaesthetist take to avoid peripheral nerve injuries in patients undergoing general or local anaesthesia? Describe the aetiology and types of lesions which may occur.

OUTLINE PLAN

Lesion
neuropraxia, axonotmesis, neurotmesis

Causes (with examples)
stretch
compression
direct (needle) injury

For each example
worst position — best position
neurological result
padding and precautions

Particular problems
arm out on board
head-down position
make note on chart

This question is phrased oddly and may lead candidates to write an unbalanced answer if they follow the sequence of the question. It is easier to answer by describing the cause of the various lesions before the steps taken to avoid the injuries arising. Suggested opening sentences:

Nerve injuries are classified as neuropraxia, axonotmesis, and neurotmesis.

The usual way in which nerves are damaged in the operating theatre is by direct mechanical trauma.

Damage to peripheral nerves is important because it is nearly always preventable.

Peripheral nerve damage is a common source of medicolegal problems arising from anaesthetic practice.

The first sentence provides an initial structure: the first topic of the full answer will describe what each term means. There is nothing wrong with it but the other, more general, sentences have more impact by showing a wider appreciation of the question. Sentence two shows that the candidate knows the usual cause of trouble; sentences three and four show that the candidate can think beyond the question.

Whatever the opening sentence, the best way to start the main answer is with a description of what happens at the level of the nerve trunk and fibre.

Lesion
neuropraxia, axonotmesis, neurotmesis
mechanism, histology, recovery

The trick now is how to avoid the repetition that is almost bound to occur if you work through a list of peripheral nerves, giving the causes of the problems and listing the precautions you would take. Instead, work through the causes and precautions, using the peripheral nerves as examples.

Causes
stretch
compression
    table and attachments
    tourniquet
    mask and harness
direct (needle) injury
    physical
        during IV or IM injection
        during nerve block injection
    chemical
(indirect injury: chemical)

For each example
worst position — best position
neurological result of damage
padding and other precautions

Working through the first list, giving examples and keeping the second list in mind, will allow you to give a good review of the main problems. Your examples should be nerves that are commonly damaged: wrist drop caused by compression of the radial nerve against the edge of a metal screen is a better example than sensory loss in the perineum caused by compression of the pudendal nerve against the ischial tuberosity. Although any nerve may be damaged by wayward needles, the best examples are the commonest: median at the elbow during intravenous injection and sciatic in the buttock during intramuscular injection.

Indirect, chemical injury is in brackets because this refers to trichloroethylene and its reaction with soda lime, which is now really only of historical interest. It is worth a sentence, but no-one will fail for omitting it.

A last section dealing with two particularly risky circumstances allows you to bring everything together:

Particular problems
> arm out on board
>> brachial plexus, ulnar nerve, radial nerve
>> optimal position, padding
> head-down position
>> brachial plexus and shoulder supports
>> and lithotomy: straps and nerves at ankle & knee
> make note on chart

It is a good idea to note the position of the arms on the anaesthetic chart. Writing this in your answer will round the essay off nicely, particularly if your first sentence referred to medicolegal problems.

Description of damage to the spinal cord and nerve roots should not be included in this question. Nor should blocks with neurolytic agents, used in pain clinics.

4-13 What are the causes of abnormal cardiac rhythm arising during anaesthesia? How may they be managed?

OUTLINE PLAN

Patient factors
> pre-existing cardiac disease
> electrolyte disturbances
> endocrine
> drugs

Anaesthetic factors
> errors
> drugs
> other

central line irritation
temperature

Surgical factors

stimulation/light anaesthesia
exogenous adrenaline
diathermy with pacemaker

Management

diagnosis
assessment
remove factors
treat
sinus bradycardia
sinus tachycardia
atrial tachycardia
ventricular ectopic beats
ventricular tachycardia or fibrillation
heart block

Possible opening sentences:

The causes of arrhythmias arising during anaesthesia may be divided into three main groups: patient factors, anaesthetic factors and surgical factors.

The most common arrhythmias arising during surgery are nodal rhythm and sinus bradycardia.

Arrhythmias during surgery are not uncommon, and usually require no management beyond checking that something, such as hypercapnia, has not been overlooked.

Arrhythmias during surgery are not uncommon and usually benign, but unless the anaesthetist has a scheme of management there is the danger that the more sinister causes of arrhythmias may be overlooked.

The first sentence gives the structure of the essay; the second tells the examiner that you realize common things occur commonly; the third gives clinical immediacy but may convey a sense of complacency; the last is the best. Without a scheme, there is also the danger of giving drugs unnecessarily, but adding this makes the sentence too long.

Patient factors

pre-existing cardiac disease
ischaemia
re-entrant circuits
electrolyte disturbances
acidosis

> endocrine
> drugs

'Drugs' needs expansion. Beware of too much detail about things like arrhythmias secondary to thyroid dysfunction; they would be unlikely to arise *during* anaesthesia now that patients are almost always rendered euthyroid preoperatively.

Anaesthetic factors

> errors
>> hypoxia, hypercapnia
> drugs
>> inhalational agents
>> muscle relaxants
>> local anaesthetic overdose
>> vasoactive drugs

'Errors' comes first because it should be the first thought of the anaesthetist when an arrhythmia is detected.

Suxamethonium is the only relaxant that *causes* bradycardia, although, because of lack of vagolysis, bradycardia is common when atracurium or vecuronium is used. 'Vasoactive drugs' is intended to include atropine.

> other
>> central line irritation
>> temperature

Both hypothermia and malignant hyperpyrexia cause arrhythmias.

Surgical factors

> stimulation/light anaesthesia
>> examples
> exogenous adrenaline
> diathermy with pacemaker

Good examples of surgically induced arrhythmias are the bradycardia caused by peritoneal stretching and the ventricular ectopics that occur during the extraction of wisdom teeth under halothane breathed spontaneously.

Management

> diagnosis
> assessment
>> ?haemodynamic compromise
> remove factors
> treat
>> sinus bradycardia
>> sinus tachycardia
>> atrial tachycardia

ventricular ectopic beats
ventricular tachycardia or fibrillation
heart block

To avoid repetition, you may prefer to discuss each arrhythmia and its management under an appropriate earlier section.

It is more important to describe the principles of treatment than the specific drug therapy for every possible arrhythmia. Arrhythmias need treatment only if there is significant haemodynamic disturbance (as can occur with a supraventricular tachycardia) or if there might be such disturbance eventually (for instance with multifocal ventricular ectopics developing into fibrillation). During anaesthesia, it is often better *not* to treat, particularly with long-acting drugs that might upset the later management of the patient. The examiners will be more impressed by a careful discussion of how you *decide* to treat, than by a list of drugs.

For completeness, you should include asystole and electromechanical dissociation, although they warrant little discussion except for possible causes, more especially of electromechanical dissociation. This is a question in which it is easy to get sidetracked and ignore clinical realities. You could write half a page describing the treatment of ventricular fibrillation — but how often does that occur *during anaesthesia*? Except during cardiac surgery, it is most likely to occur as a terminal event in a desperately ill patient — when the correct management might be to do nothing.

Remember that ST and T wave changes are not in themselves arrhythmias.

4-14 Discuss the use of the oesophagus as a site for monitoring during anaesthesia.

OUTLINE PLAN

Oesophageal stethoscope
    description
    cardiopulmonary monitoring
       air embolism

Temperature measurement
    relation to core temperature

Depth of anaesthesia
    motility

Cardiac monitoring
    transoesophageal echocardiography

Opening sentences

The oesophageal stethoscope and temperature probe are already widely used, and there is now much research into the transoesophageal measurement of cardiac output as well as the possible measurement of anaesthetic depth from oesophageal motility.

The oesophagus is a convenient route of access to the thorax that allows easy and effectively non-invasive monitoring of basic cardiopulmonary function.

Some anaesthetists looking after paediatric and neurosurgical cases use oesophageal monitoring routinely, and it seems likely that this useful approach will become more common.

This is a general essay, more appropriate at Part 3, that allows those candidates who have read more than the basic facts to impress the examiners. Obey the general rule of going from the familiar to the experimental: start with the oesophageal stethoscope and work through to monitors of cardiac function.

Oesophageal stethoscope
   description
   breath sounds
   heart sounds
      air embolism
   advantages

The simple oesophageal stethoscope can be turned into a more sophisticated (and expensive) device by incorporating a thermistor and electrocardiogram leads. Do not get sidetracked by these yet; deal first with the simple, inexpensive and invaluable plain oesophageal stethoscope. Do not forget the real advantage that the anaesthetist is fixed to the patient by a length of plastic tubing.

Temperature measurement
      why useful (brief)
   description
   relation to core temperature
   which patients especially?

If you know the physics behind the measurement, a sentence or two is not out of place; but physics would not be expected in the answer. What will be expected is a discussion of what the oesophageal temperature means, and what the advantages and disadvantages are of using this as a measure of body temperature.

Half your answer should be of the fairly routine uses of the oesophagus in monitoring. The order in which you tackle the second, more speculative, half depends on which of the topics you know most about: the better known should come first.

Depth of anaesthesia

motility
    spontaneous and provoked contractions
current state of practical application

The first question of this chapter was about the monitoring of depth of anaesthesia (see p. 69). There is time in this question for only an outline of what you might have been able to write for that.

Cardiac monitoring

electrocardiography
transoesophageal echocardiography
    cardiac output
    regional wall motion
practical application

The equipment for measuring beat-by-beat cardiac output in this way is certain to become more reliable, smaller and less expensive with time. But before you start extolling the value of having this information during *routine* perioperative monitoring, ask yourself what you would do with the information, and whether you could act upon it sensibly.

The measurement of pressures in the thoracic oesophagus in the course of measuring pulmonary compliance should not be discussed.

4-15 Discuss the causes and management of postoperative hypoxia.

OUTLINE PLAN

Hypoventilation

airway obstruction
central depression
residual neuromuscular blockade
other causes of ventilatory embarrassment

Diffusion hypoxia

Shivering

Ventilation/perfusion mismatch

mechanism
    functional residual capacity and closing volume
    dependent atelectasis

Treatment

underlying cause
oxygen therapy
    variable performance devices

```
fixed performance devices
consider (re)intubation, further measures
```

A stock question suitable for both Part 1 and Part 3 of the examination; and, for candidates at Part 3, one that relies heavily on the physiology learned for Part 2. Any anaesthetist failing to give a satisfactory answer to this question would deservedly fail the examination. However, even the best of candidates can fail if they overlook a whole subsection of the answer — and that is easy to do with a question like this. It seems so straightforward, indeed it is so straightforward, that there is the temptation to ignore the need to write a plan. *Always* write a plan.

Possible opening sentences:

> Postoperative hypoxia is both common and important and the increasing availability of pulse oximeters has made us realize just how common it is.

> A degree of postoperative hypoxia should be regarded as inevitable and every patient recovering from general anaesthesia must breathe an oxygen-enriched gas mixture to minimize the risk of complications of severe hypoxia.

> Postoperative hypoxia may be associated with myocardial ischaemia, arrhythmias, hypertension and cerebral ischaemia, all of which adversely affect postoperative outcome.

The first two sentences are better than the third, which, although it appears to be punchy and to warn of the dangers of hypoxia, is both too obvious when extreme (hypoxia damages cerebral cells and causes arrhythmias) but is uncertain when less extreme (do we have evidence that lesser degrees of hypoxia, detectable by pulse oximetry, affect outcome?). The third sentence is also less good at leading into the start of the answer, which should be dealing with physiology not pathology.

Hypoxia is classically put into four headings: hypoxic, anaemic, stagnant and histotoxic. These are not so useful in a discussion of postoperative hypoxia. There is a tendency to write first about diffusion hypoxia, but the commonest cause of hypoxia is simple hypoventilation, and that should be described first.

Hypoventilation
```
airway obstruction
central depression
residual neuromuscular blockade
sleep apnoea
```

These are three topics that must be discussed at length. What exactly is obstructing the airway? Describe the way you would teach a recovery nurse to clear the airway. Give details of the drugs that cause central depression of ventilation; do not forget hypocapnia. Remember that residual neuromuscular blockade affects ventilation by adding to airway obstruction more than by a primary failure to move enough air.

At the time of writing, sleep apnoea is topical. It is more important in the days rather than hours after operation (see below).

> other causes of ventilatory embarrassment
> > pain
> > diaphragmatic splinting
> > (rare) preoperative neuromuscular disease and electrolyte
> > > abnormalities
> > (do not forget) bronchospasm, pneumothorax
>
> **Diffusion hypoxia**
> > mechanism
> > significance
>
> **Increased consumption**
> > shivering

Where appropriate in these sections of the answer, you can simply write that 'Oxygen should be given by mask . . .'. The later part of the answer will include a section on the principles of masks and oxygen therapy so there is no need to keep repeating what type of mask and what concentration of oxygen you would use.

> **Ventilation/perfusion mismatch and increased shunt**
> > mechanism (physiology)
> > cause (always)
> > > functional residual capacity and closing volume
> > > dependent atelectasis
> > > > exaggerated with one-lung anaesthesia
> > > hypoxic vasoconstrictive reflex
> > cause (often after abdominal surgery)
> > > infection
> > cause (rarely)
> > > cardiac failure, overtransfusion
> > > aspiration
>
> **Treatment**
> > underlying cause
> > oxygen therapy
> > > physiology in hypoventilation
> > > physiology in $\dot{V}/\dot{Q}$ disturbance

When you come to write the full answer, specific treatments of underlying causes (for example, naloxone to reverse opioids) may be better described earlier because they will only take a sentence or two.

variable performance devices
   mode of action
   types
fixed performance devices
   mode of action
   types
if (rare) not sufficient
   consider (re)intubation, further measures

Most patients will be well served by a Hudson or MC mask or similar. Do not give the examiner the impression that you do not consider these devices satisfactory because the actual value of the inspired oxygen is unknown.

Patients with pre-existing respiratory disease are particularly at risk of hypoxia after operations. You can make comments to this effect at appropriate points in the answer. Do not be sidetracked into too much discussion of, for example, chronic obstructive airways disease. The question as asked is a general question that demands a general answer; and the physiology underlying the hypoxia of chronic bronchitic patients, though exaggerated, is the same as that for other patients.

A more difficult problem when considering this question is whether 'postoperative hypoxia' includes the first few *days* after operation. All patients are at risk of severe hypoxia in the first few minutes to hours after operation; rather fewer are at risk of hypoxia after that, and it is uncertain what the ill-effects of this usually less severe hypoxia are. It is probably better to put in comments about longer-lasting hypoxia at appropriate points in your answer rather than having a specific section on it.

4-16 Discuss the relative advantages and disadvantages of different ways by which opioids may be given for postoperative pain relief.

OUTLINE PLAN

Intramuscular (IM)

drugs used
on demand: for and against
regular: for and against

Intravenous (IV)

incremental
infusion
patient-controlled analgesia (PCA)
   description
   for and against

Peridural
>(spinal)
>epidural catheter
>drugs
>for and against

Other routes

An obvious opening sentence is to give a list, but it is better to list just the common routes rather than all the possibilities.

Postoperative opioids are commonly given by the intramuscular, intravenous, and epidural routes.

The historical approach is a good one.

Opioids are given traditionally by intramuscular injection, but this has disadvantages that have led to the development of other techniques.

After the introduction, the descriptive part of the answer must start with intramuscular papaveretum given on demand, because that is still the most common method — although morphine may come to replace it as the most used postoperative opioid if papaveretum is confirmed as genotoxic.

Intramuscular (IM)
>drugs used
>general disadvantage: pain on injection
>on demand
>>for: easy, inexpensive
>>>no sudden side-effects
>>>nurses can assess
>>against: delay
>>>fluctuating plasma concentrations
>>>side-effects, drowsiness
>regularly
>>for: no delay
>>against: uncertainty of correct dose

IM is an acceptable abbreviation for intramuscular. Do not introduce the IM route merely to dismiss it as unsatisfactory, in favour of more sophisticated techniques. It is a technique that gives many patients excellent relief of pain.

When discussing the drugs, papaveretum is the standard (do not write Omnopon™) and none of the others have any real advantage but write of one or two others if you wish, particularly those of which you have experience. This is more appropriate for Part 3.

Intravenous (IV)
>general advantage: no pain on injection

    incremental
      for: can titrate
      against: takes time
        practical only in recovery room
    infusion:
      for: continuous analgesia
      against: needs separate IV cannula
        choosing rate
        cumulation
    patient-controlled analgesia (PCA)
      description
      for: no delay, continuous analgesia
        (but sleep)
        relatively safe
      against: design must be made fail-safe
        expensive

You will need to write a sentence or two of description of PCA, particularly the ways that the machines are set up to prevent overdose. PCA, especially with or without background infusion, is a topic of debate.

Peridural

    (spinal)
    epidural catheter
    drugs
    for: excellent pain relief
       (especially plus local anaesthetic)
    against: takes time to insert
      (usual complications)
      late respiratory depression

Epidural opioids are even more a topic of debate. Remember that no-one knows the relative risks of respiratory side-effects of opioids given epidurally or intramuscularly; and some people think that giving opioids by the epidural route is merely a complicated way of giving an intravenous infusion. At Part 1 you should mention the technique if you know about it, and give more detail if you are familiar with it. At Part 3 you will be expected to be familiar with it, and you should know about the controversies.

Note that the question asks only about opioids, so a brief mention of local anaesthetics, combined with opioids, is all that is needed.

Other routes

    oral
    sublingual
    rectal
    transdermal

These routes are of limited use postoperatively, and could probably be omitted from an answer at Part 1. You would not fail the examination if you did not mention them at Part 3, but a complete answer includes a discussion of them.

CHAPTER 5

Anaesthesia for specific diseases or conditions

INTRODUCTION

We will consider, first, by looking in a more general way at the question planned in 5-1, the overall strategy for tackling this type of question — a standard question at both Parts 1 and 3: how would you anaesthetize a patient with a specific disease? These are the easiest questions to plan for in advance.

Q   Discuss the anaesthetic management of a grossly obese patient presenting for elective intra-abdominal surgery.

The first plan below is a universal scheme. Specific questions, such as the one asked here about obesity, will require plans modified from the basic pattern, with certain topics emphasized or omitted according to the disease, the precise wording of the question, and your detailed knowledge.

Preoperatively
    expected problems
        because of patient
        because of operation
        because of circumstances
    assessment
        history
        examination
        investigations, with reasons
    preparation of patient
        treatment
            postponement/cancellation
        resuscitation
    premedication
        psychological
        pharmacological

The operation
    general, regional, or combined?
    induction: specific problems and aims

                  technique, drugs, airway, intubation
                  monitoring
            maintenance: problems and aims
                  positioning
                  drugs
                     hypnosis, relaxation, analgesia
                  ventilation
                  monitoring
                  fluids
            reversal: yes or no
                  drugs

Postoperatively: specific problems and aims

   disposal
      ward/ICU?
   continuing management
      analgesia (method, drugs)
      fluids
   instructions to nursing staff

Follow-up: e.g. counselling

5-1   Discuss the anaesthetic management of a grossly obese patient presenting for elective intra-abdominal surgery.

OUTLINE PLAN

Preoperatively

   expected problems
      anatomy
      respiration
      cardiovascular
      aspiration risk
      other associated disease
      pharmacokinetics
   premedication and adjuvants

The operation

   general ± regional
   induction: rapid sequence
      monitoring
   maintenance: drugs
   reversal: yes or no

Postoperatively: ward/ICU?

   especially analgesia
   mobility

The question asks about the management of a *grossly obese* patient presenting for *elective* surgery that is *intra-abdominal*. If you find yourself writing, 'If the patient is not too obese ...', 'When patients like this present as emergencies ...', or 'For operations on the extremities ...', you are getting off the point.

An opening sentence on the lines of 'There will be physiological, pharmacological and anatomical considerations ...' is satisfactory but you are going to have to define gross obesity at some stage and in the opening sentence is a good place:

> There are a number of definitions of morbid obesity: one is more than 45 kg above ideal weight, another is double the ideal weight. A man of 5'8" who weighed around 140 kg would be in this category.

Giving an example is repetition but gives a better mental image of a patient. The plan can be a modification of the general one presented above, for which an outline with some specific detail is:

Preoperatively
> expected problems
> anatomy
>> veins, airway, lifting, positioning
>> regional blocks
>> external chest compression
> respiration
>> compliance
>> ventilation/perfusion mismatch
>> carbon dioxide response
> cardiovascular
>> hypertension
>> ischaemic heart disease
> aspiration risk
> other associated disease
>> (endocrine obesity)
>> diabetes
>> osteoarthritis
>> liver disease
>> clotting
> pharmacokinetics
> psychological makeup

This already looks an awful lot, but in shorthand it would take little time:

Preop
> problems:

anat: IVI aw heavy limbs LA CPR??
resp: Paw $\dot{V}/\dot{Q}$ CO_2
CVS: +BP IHD
HH
other: (rare) diab OA LFTs DVT
pharmkin
psych

This first section is important because you will already have dealt with most of the important principles of later management, for instance the problems of ventilation, and you will be able to refer back when appropriate. There is a lot of detail to write, which means that, unless the question states specifically that the patient is diabetic or hypertensive, there is no need to discuss your management of these conditions once you have made the statement that they are more common in the grossly obese.

Having made this list, the section on preoperative assessment can be short: a sentence that your assessment would be directed to evaluating these problems, and what non-routine investigations you would require. The plan then continues:

premedication
anxiolysis, antacid, heparin

The operation:

general ± regional (?heparin)
induction: rapid sequence
monitoring
?invasive blood pressure
maintenance: drugs
which volatile?
which relaxant?
reversal: yes or no

Postoperatively: ward/ICU?

continuing management
analgesia (method, drugs)
get mobile
physiotherapy

This later section of the plan follows the standard plan quite closely. The main danger is of your answer being a list of *could do this and might do that*. There is no one correct anaesthetic for this patient. Tell the examiner what you would do and why: whether you choose temazepam, thoracic epidural, minimal isoflurane, no opioid, and then extubate and observe; or papaveretum and hyoscine, fentanyl, enflurane as indicated, and ventilate overnight on the intensive care unit.

5-2 Discuss the anaesthetic management of a patient with a known family history of malignant hyperpyrexia for emergency laparotomy.

OUTLINE PLAN

Preoperative assessment
  including current clinical state

Premedication

Triggering drugs/safe drugs

Preparation of the theatre

Anaesthetic technique
  induction
  maintenance
    drugs

Monitoring for a crisis
  clinical signs
  monitoring

If suspected
  investigations
  action

Postoperatively
  intensive care
  counselling

This question is more likely at Part 3; an anaesthetist who has not yet passed Part 1 would be expected to contact a more senior anaesthetist before giving an anaesthetic to a patient known to be at risk of malignant hyperpyrexia. However, any anaesthetist must be able to cope at least initially with a patient who shows signs of the syndrome unexpectedly so the condition comes firmly into the syllabus at both Parts.

There is no better opening sentence than a brief definition of the condition.

> Malignant hyperpyrexia (MH) is a potentially fatal disorder in which extreme stress or some common anaesthetic drugs trigger severe metabolic disturbances combined with rigidity of skeletal muscles.

MH is an accepted abbreviation.

The first paragraph can be finished off with a second sentence:

> The basis of successful anaesthetic management is the avoidance of precipitating factors and the rapid and appropriate treatment of a crisis if it occurs.

This patient must be treated as positive for malignant hyperpyrexia. There is no time for any tests so there is no point in detailed descriptions of them in your answer. The question specifies a known family history, but not which members of the family. This gives you the opportunity for a *brief* summary of the method of inheritance and who might have been tested, and a statement about diagnostic muscle biopsy and its reliability.

The question specifies 'emergency laparotomy', so do not forget to include a simple description of the routine anaesthetic management of the acute abdomen.

Preoperative assessment
    previous anaesthetics
    family history
    current clinical state

Premedication
    sedation
    prophylaxis against acid aspiration
    dantrolene

You are not given any information about the diagnosis so make only general statements about any necessary preoperative treatment. For example, 'An intravenous infusion should be started and adequate fluid given before induction,' is sufficient; there is no need for detail about severity of dehydration and hypovolaemia, consideration of what type of fluid to give, or what you would do for perforated ulcer, large bowel obstruction, or any other specific condition.

Give drugs and doses of premedicant drugs. Details of pretreatment with dantrolene will not be expected for Part 1. Dantrolene can be given orally or intravenously — but this patient has an acute abdomen and it will not impress the examiners to suggest oral treatment.

Triggering drugs/safe drugs

Every anaesthetist needs to know a list of safe drugs for conditions well known to cause anaesthetic problems, of which malignant hyperpyrexia and porphyria are the best known. You do not need to give a list of all known possible triggers and all recognized safe drugs. This is an emergency laparotomy so you must stress the avoidance of suxamethonium, and you must write about the difficulties of not being able to use volatile agents.

Preparation of the theatre
    (routine check)
    vapour-free anaesthetic machine
    cooling aids
    drugs

Anaesthetic technique
    induction
        with non-depolarizing agent

> awake intubation?
> maintenance
> drugs
> + epidural?

'Routine check' is in brackets because no more than, 'After a routine check of the equipment . . .,' is required. You can list the cooling aids and drugs at this stage, or you can leave that until the section of the essay in which you will be describing their use (see below).

Cricoid pressure is an effective manoeuvre: provided that there is no suggestion of a difficult intubation, there is no reason why a large dose of vecuronium will not enable satisfactorily early protection of the airway. Propofol is safe and an infusion is an easy way of providing anaesthesia without the need for a volatile agent.

Monitoring for a crisis

> clinical signs
> temperature
> capnography
> electrocardiogram
> oximetry

If suspected:

> investigations
>> take arterial blood sample for acid-base status and
>> potassium

Describe the changes, what causes them, and in what order they would be likely to occur. Clinical signs, as always, should be mentioned before electronic monitors, even though the first suspicion may be because of a rising end-tidal carbon dioxide concentration or a rising temperature. Further blood tests, for muscle enzymes, lactate and myoglobin, for instance, are not worth writing about, not because they do not change but because they are of no help in the immediate management.

If suspected:

> action
>> adequate gas exchange
>> dantrolene
>> lines and tubes
>> aggressive cooling
>> treat acidosis and hyperkalaemia
>> fluids
>> arrhythmias
>> intensive care postoperatively

Postoperatively

> counselling, testing

All these topics need considerable expansion, with firm details of your management. The patient's life depends on what you do here and — for this question as asked — these details are more important than describing the process of testing or details of the inheritance of the condition. 'Adequate gas exchange' means providing a suitable concentration of oxygen to prevent hypoxia and an adequate minute volume to prevent hypercapnia.

The essay can be rounded off with a short paragraph about counselling.

5-3 Six weeks after a major myocardial infarction a 58-year-old man requires urgent laparotomy. Discuss your anaesthetic management.

OUTLINE PLAN

Principles: care with blood pressure and heart rate

Preoperative assessment

operation, recent history
cardiovascular status
concurrent problems

Premedication

Induction

think 1. cardiovascular system
      2. emergency abdominal surgery
monitoring, drugs, technique

Maintenance

drugs, ventilation, monitoring, fluids

Anticipated problems and treatments

tachycardia, bradycardia
hypertension, hypotension
ischaemic changes
arrhythmias, heart block
cardiac failure

Postoperatively

analgesia, ?ventilation
clear plan

A 'major myocardial infarction' implies that there was or still is heart failure or serious arrhythmias. Any discussion of minor infarction, which will not have affected the cardiovascular reserve of the patient, is not relevant.

Opening sentences: the second is better:

A patient who has an anaesthetic and surgery six weeks after a myocardial infarction has a greatly increased risk of re-infarcting in the postoperative period.

A patient who has had a myocardial infarction six weeks previously is at risk of heart failure, heart block, arrhythmias and re-infarction.

Your plan should then state the principles of your technique before following a chronological pattern.

Principles:
avoid extremes of blood pressure and heart rate

Preoperative assessment:
operative diagnosis
what happened six weeks previously
current cardiovascular status:
    failure, rhythm, drugs
any concurrent problem
adjust treatment if indicated
    ?pace

The section on principles should include a short paragraph on the underlying physiology, i.e. the maintenance of coronary blood flow and the balance between oxygen supply and metabolic demand.

The best known prognostic indicator is the Goldman index. By all means discuss this, but you must discuss it in the context of this patient, who is already at risk by fulfilling three of the criteria. Candidates have a tendency to go into automatic mode, listing all the criteria whatever the circumstances. You must show you are thinking appropriately: one of the criteria is *age over 70 years*; this man is 58.

Premedication
?analgesia

Induction
two aspects: cardiovascular
    emergency abdominal surgery
monitoring
    ?how much, ?in theatre
choice of drugs
technique

Premedication is not an important part of the management of this patient.

The monitoring you require, and whether you require all or some of it during induction, will depend on the state of the patient and the proposed operation. The approach to this man if he is in overt heart failure and has a suspected ruptured abdominal aneurysm will be different from the approach if he has no heart failure and a perforated duodenal ulcer. It is obviously not possible to list all the possible combinations of condition and operation; what the examiners want is a reasoned argument with examples of what, in practice, you would do.

Urgent implies laparotomy as an emergency, with precautions for the full stomach. This is not a question that is asking for detail about the full stomach, so 'rapid sequence induction with preoxygenation and cricoid pressure' is sufficient.

Maintenance

opioids, volatile agents
ventilation
monitoring
fluids

Anticipated problems:

tachycardia
bradycardia
hypertension
hypotension
ischaemic changes
arrhythmias
   heart block
cardiac failure

This is the most important part of the answer. You must give a confident scheme of management, remembering that there is no single, correct technique. Epidurals are not appropriate for a possibly unstable patient having urgent surgery.

Postoperatively

?elective ventilation
analgesia
monitoring
clear plan

You need to discuss what would make you elect to ventilate the patient on the intensive care unit or, say, observe overnight in a high dependency unit or recovery ward. It is important that the anaesthetists and surgeons have a clear plan of what to do if there are early postoperative complications as the plan will depend on the surgical prognosis.

5-4 In what way are the consequences of renal failure of importance to the anaesthetist?

OUTLINE PLAN

Physiology:

fluids and electrolytes

cardiovascular system
respiratory system
nervous system
haematology
bones
immunology

Pharmacology

premedicants, induction agents, relaxants
volatile agents

Practical

veins, fistulae, postoperative analgesia

Beware of the opening sentence:

Renal failure has a number of important implications for the anaesthetist.

The examiners would not have asked the question unless this was so. A better option is to use the opening sentence to give the basic structure of your answer:

Amongst the many consequences of renal failure are problems of fluid and electrolyte balance, coexisting cardiovascular disease, haematological disturbance, concurrent drug therapy and altered pharmacokinetics.

This sentence starts '*Amongst* the many . . .' so that it is purposely not complete, which allows you later to discuss, for instance, bone disease without feeling you have to modify the opening sentence.

Another possibility is:

Many of the problems of disordered physiology that occur with renal failure are much less of a problem to anaesthetists now that dialysis is effective and donated kidneys can be kept for longer periods, and often the biggest practical difficulty for anaesthetists is finding a suitable vein.

This type of sentence shows the examiners that you know what is important and that you are able to do more than merely regurgitate a couple of pages of textbook detail about renal failure.

This is a difficult question to plan, because patients with renal failure are such a heterogeneous group. For instance, should the answer discuss patients with a working transplant, who could be considered fit and healthy and do not really have renal failure any longer?

The best approach is probably by systems, with practical details added where relevant.

Physiology

fluids

    distribution, plasma proteins
electrolytes
    esp. potassium and acid–base
        treatment for hyperkalaemia
cardiovascular system
    hypertension
        drugs
    heart failure
    pericardial effusions
respiratory system
    susceptible to infection
nervous system
    uraemic encephalopathy
    autonomic neuropathy
haematology
    anaemia
    platelet dysfunction
    heparin for dialysis
bones
    calcium
immunology
    prone to infection
        (immunosuppression for transplant)
    hep B and HIV

The question asks specifically for the consequences for the anaesthetist, so, for each sub-heading, write why that particular physiological disturbance has implications for the anaesthetist.

Pharmacology
    premedicants
    induction agents
    relaxants
        suxamethonium and potassium
        non-depolarizers
    volatile agents
        fluoride ion

There are many pharmacological effects of renal failure; the topic itself would make a good question at either Part 1 or Part 3. With the question asked here, there will not be time to go into great detail and you should concentrate on the important practical problems. This gives a good opportunity to impress the examiners that you know what is important. Discussing thiopentone, it is all too easy to get bogged down in theoretical considerations of protein binding (which may increase the sensitivity of the patient) while ignoring the reality that increased cardiac output secondary to anaemia may mean that a larger dose than normal is needed for induction. Similarly, a long paragraph detailing the renal excretion of all the non-depolarizing neuromuscular blockers is unnecessary; the important practical point is that the newer relaxants have virtually eliminated problems of prolonged block or recurarization.

Practical

veins
  using dialysis lines
fistulae
  protection
postoperative analgesia

If you have not already done so earlier in the essay, one way of rounding off would be a short paragraph about the range of patients who present to the anaesthetist with renal failure. You cannot mention every possibility, but for contrast you could include the patient with a working transplant presenting incidentally for surgery, the patient acutely ill who needs a transplant nephrectomy, and the patient with no visible veins in whom the surgeons wish to fashion a fistula.

5-5 Discuss the anaesthetic management of a patient with severe chronic obstructive airways disease presenting for elective abdominal surgery.

OUTLINE PLAN

Definitions

Assessment

  history, examination, investigations

Preparation

  get as well as possible

Perioperative

  premedication, induction, maintenance, ventilation
    monitoring
  possible problems

Recovery

Postoperatively

The three important words to underline are *severe*, *abdominal* and *elective*. Patients with severe chronic obstructive airways disease *will have* an increased $PaCO_2$ *and* a decreased PaO_2; discussion of anaesthesia for patients with one or the other is not needed. Similarly, it is all too easy to find yourself writing: 'If such a patient presents as an emergency . . .' or 'If relaxation is needed . . .'. When these patients present as emergencies it can be quite a clinical challenge, but on this occasion the examiners have not asked about it. Similarly, abdominal surgery requires relaxed muscles.

The opening sentence should define what is meant by severe disease, enumerate the main perioperative problems, or quote briefly from one of the studies that have tried to relate perioperative tests of respiratory function to postoperative morbidity. Beware of 'Patients with severe chronic obstructive airways disease present a difficult challenge to the anaesthetist', which tells the examiner nothing.

> The main problems that the anaesthetist must consider in patients with severe chronic obstructive airways disease (COAD) are excessive production of sputum (with the increased risk of postoperative atelectasis and chest infection), airways obstruction, the loss of ventilatory response to carbon dioxide, and dependence on hypoxic drive.

This is a long sentence, but the question is a big one and there will not be time to go into any detail of the aetiology or pathology of the condition. Perhaps the next sentence should mention the range of disease: the idea of pink puffers and blue bloaters. The first sentence, being a summary of the main problems, allows you to get on with the anaesthetic management, which covers the whole perioperative course: the plan must start with preoperative assessment. COAD is a recognized abbreviation but you should still define it the first time you use it.

Assessment
history, examination
investigations: especially ECG, CXR, spirometry
  (with bronchodilators)

There is no need to list absolutely every symptom, sign and investigation. Do not forget assessment of respiratory function at the bedside; timing a vital capacity breath and the duration of breath holding are useful. Almost everyone knows of the test in which the patient tries to blow out a lighted match, but this is not a practical test (how many people carry around matches?) and examinations are about practical anaesthesia not what candidates can remember from outdated textbooks.

Preparation
timing
smoking
infection
bronchospasm
physiotherapy
cor pulmonale

These patients should have their operation when they are in as good condition as possible. *Timing* covers two things: the time of year when they should be admitted; and how long before surgery they should be admitted to allow adequate treatment.

The plan now moves into the operative phase: be decisive; say which drugs you would use and why.

Premedication: benzodiazepine or none

Induction: etomidate, fentanyl, vecuronium

Maintenance: halothane, ?epidural

Ventilation: flow generator, keep $PaCO_2$ at pre-induction value, avoid high airway pressure, allow prolonged expiration

Monitoring: capnography and pulse oximetry particularly useful

This plan is not necessarily the only correct anaesthetic technique; but whichever you choose must be justified, even if the justification is to write that whether drug A or drug B is used there is likely to be little difference in outcome.

Problems and treatment: bronchospasm, sputum, (rarely: pneumothorax)

Recovery: consider elective postoperative ventilation, better not lying flat

Postoperatively
analgesia
oxygen — doxapram? — nasal CPAP?
bronchodilators, antibiotics, physiotherapy
care with fluids

5-6 Describe the anaesthetic management of a patient with a cardiac pacemaker undergoing transurethral resection of the prostate.

OUTLINE PLAN

Preoperative problems
assess patient
assess pacemaker
premedication

Operation
spinal or general?
cardiovascular stability during TURP
pacemaker

   fixed output
    advantages of spinal or GA
    central venous pressure line?
Diathermy and pacemaker
  use of diathermy
  monitoring
  pacemaker to fixed mode?
   (microshock)
If pacing fails
Postop
  recovery

'Anaesthetic management' includes preoperative assessment, which is particularly important in patients with a pacemaker. They are usually old and have concurrent disease, if only because most rhythm disturbances in the elderly are secondary to ischaemic heart disease. Do not, however, spend too much time on the detail of how you might treat preoperative problems.

Patients having a prostatic operation are themselves, even without a pacemaker, old and likely to be ill. Again, you must not concentrate too much on aspects of the operation irrelevant to a consideration of the pacemaker. Your answer must not be to the question 'Describe the anaesthetic management of a patient undergoing transurethral resection of the prostate' with consideration of the pacemaker tacked on; you simply will not have time for that. What this means is that you must select those aspects of TURP that are of particular relevance when the patient has a pacemaker. Thus, although you must obviously mention TUR syndrome, you do not need to discuss it and its management in detail.

Possible opening sentences:

> Patients with pacemakers are at risk of microshock and of interference with the function of the pacemaker if diathermy is used during the operation.

This sentence is an example of how to start an essay with entirely the wrong emphasis. Not only does it emphasize the pacemaker and not the patient, but microshock — a small theoretical risk — is mentioned before an important practical one.

> Patients with prostatic enlargement and a pacemaker are often old and ill, and intercurrent disease may be as much of a worry to the anaesthetist as the pacemaker itself.

> Patients with a pacemaker face risks during surgery because the resulting fixed heart rate limits haemodynamic compensation and because diathermy can interfere with the function of pacemakers.

Either of these sentences is good, though the first may lead the candidate to write too much about intercurrent disease. The second states the most common risks plainly.

Preoperative problems
　assess patient
　　cardiac disease
　　renal disease
　　other
　assess pacemaker
　　type
　　　fixed, demand
　　function
　premedication

Make brief statements of the likely intercurrent diseases and the necessary investigations. Whether the pacemaker is working properly is more important than knowing the exact mode of its operation.

Operation
　spinal or general?

This is the crux of the question. You must be able to discuss it clearly on a background of cardiovascular physiology. There is no absolutely 'correct' method of anaesthesia. If you have a preference, state it and give the examiners the reasons. The logical way to start this section is by describing how a pacemaker affects cardiovascular stability.

　cardiovascular stability during TURP
　　position
　　blood loss
　　infused fluids
　　　TUR syndrome
　pacemaker
　　fixed output
　　　advantages of spinal or GA
　　　central venous pressure line?
　your choice

You do not need to give details of spinal technique, except for drug dosage and level of block because these are important to cardiovascular stability. Give an outline of a technique for general anaesthesia; most anaesthetists would probably intubate and ventilate using a low concentration of a volatile agent.

As an example of unnecessary detail: you should mention the lithotomy position because of its effects on the cardiovascular system, but in this answer its effects on the breathing system and as a possible factor in regurgitation are irrelevant.

Diathermy and pacemaker

plate away from pacemaker
short bursts
bipolar better than unipolar
electrocardiograph should reject diathermy artefact
    pulse monitor
pacemaker to fixed mode?
    microshock

If pacing fails

isoprenaline infusion

Postop

recovery

Pulse oximeters are affected by diathermy: a finger on the pulse is a good monitor. Microshock is extremely rare, but is perhaps more likely with a temporary pacemaker that has a long wire.

Discussion of your action if the pacing fails leads back to earlier discussion of whether to insert a central venous line.

There is nothing special about the recovery phase except that you may choose to monitor the electrocardiogram, though this is not really necessary if the pacemaker has given no trouble.

5-7   Describe the perioperative management of a 13-year-old girl with acute appendicitis who is an unstable diabetic.

OUTLINE PLAN

Assessment

general
biochemical

Treatment

hyperglycaemia
ketoacidosis
timing of operation

Operative phase

anaesthetic drugs
because of appendicitis
because of diabetes
    continuing control
    caution with $P_E'CO_2$
reversal and extubation

Postoperatively
> analgesia
> control for how long?

When asked about diabetes, candidates tend to go into 'automatic mode'. They start by classifying diabetics as insulin-dependent or non-insulin-dependent, and surgery as minor, intermediate or major, routine or emergency; and continue by considering what to do with each type of diabetic for the types of surgery. This is a good way of tackling, 'Discuss the perioperative management of diabetes', but the examiners have given you precise information. Your question must concentrate on that: 13-year-olds with unstable diabetes will not be taking oral hypoglycaemics; if she is described as 'unstable' then she cannot be a newly-diagnosed, and so far untreated, diabetic.

> The management of this girl depends on the degree of instability of the diabetic state.

> This girl is likely to be dehydrated and hyperglycaemic and more generally ill than a non-diabetic with appendicitis.

> Although acute appendicitis is an emergency, the operation must be delayed until the diabetes has been brought under control.

> The first priorities with this girl are biochemical assessment, intravenous fluids, and the setting-up of an insulin infusion but, because of the risk of perforation, an operation for acute appendicitis cannot wait until diabetic control is perfect.

The first sentence is too obvious, and gives no detail at all. The second is a better general summary. The third ignores the dangers of acute appendicitis, stated explicitly in the fourth, and best, sentence.

Assessment
> general
> biochemical
>> history: normal treatment
>> investigations

Treatment
> hyperglycaemia
> ketoacidosis
>> dangers of too rapid correction
>> ?intensive care
> timing of operation
> premedication

You will need to give full details of your treatment, and comments about the range of severity expected. There is no need to write about a number of schemes, and answers that do this — 'You could do this . . .', 'Some people do that . . .' — are not as good as those that give a clear scheme: 'My preference is for a combined glucose–potassium–insulin infusion, with additional saline as required . . .'. You cannot give all possible dosages for all possible severities of condition, but you must give some examples of expected biochemical values, volumes of fluid to infuse and doses of insulin to give.

Operative phase
    anaesthetic drugs
    because of appendicitis
        rapid-sequence induction
        antibiotic prophylaxis
    because of diabetes
        continuing control: no Hartmann's
            biochemical monitoring
        caution with $P_E'CO_2$
        ?nasogastric tube
    reversal and extubation

The comment 'anaesthetic drugs' is for a sentence to the effect that no modern drugs have any effect of themselves on the diabetic state. Relative hyperventilation may be necessary to avoid dangerously low pH. The more ill the patient, the more the indication for a nasogastric tube preoperatively; otherwise consider insertion at operation.

Postoperatively:
    analgesia
    continue control
        for how long?

Your answer should not include stabilization of the diabetes once the perioperative period is over.

The question specifies a 13-year-old *girl*; make sure in such a question not to lapse into the use of the pronoun *he*.

5-8 Discuss the perioperative complications of subtotal thyroidectomy.

OUTLINE PLAN

Assessment of thyroid function
    ?further treatment
Assessment of airway
    formal vocal cord study

General assessment

Operative phase

difficult airway

equipment

spontaneous breathing or ventilate?

problems

haemostasis

arrhythmias

thyroid crisis

hypotension

Extubation and recovery

no coughing

airway

bleeding: ?tracheal compression

recurrent laryngeal nerve injury

Later complications

thyroid crisis

This is a straightforward question, which should be tackled on the standard: physiology—pathology, preoperative—peroperative—postoperative, plan. The introductory sentence should simply lead into the first phase of the answer:

Patients for subtotal thyroidectomy must have their thyroid function assessed preoperatively so that they can be given the appropriate medical treatment to make them euthyroid before surgery.

The two main concerns of the anaesthetist before subtotal thyroidectomy are thyroid function and possible respiratory obstruction.

Assessment of thyroid function

clinical

drugs

investigation

?further treatment

Assessment of airway

history

radiographs

formal vocal cord study

General assessment

Beware of statements such as 'Patients must have thoracic inlet views . . .'; there is no need if a patient is having a subtotal thyroidectomy for a simple cold nodule in a small, clinically circumscribed gland. Do not forget that the trachea can be seen on a plain chest X-ray.

Operative phase

difficult airway
   premedication
equipment: tracheal tubes
     eyes
     IV access
maintenance
   spontaneous breathing or ventilate?
problems
   haemostasis
     venous pressure
   arrhythmias
   thyroid crisis
   hypotension

Give an outline of the procedure for difficult airway. You will not impress the examiners by writing the usual 'Surgeons should stand by to perform an emergency tracheostomy' if you fail to mention that this procedure is highly dangerous — if not impossible — when the thyroid gland is enlarged.

Possible difficulties with the airway are an important consideration when thinking of premedication.

Detail of action and drugs will be needed for each of the 'problems'.

Extubation and recovery

coughing
look at cords
airway
   bleeding: ?tracheal compression
   recurrent laryngeal nerve injury
   laryngeal oedema (later)

Later complications

thyroid crisis
(hypothyroidism)

Hypothyroidism will not become apparent for some days, so is probably not a perioperative complication.

Two complications most commonly associated with thyroidectomy by anaesthetists are acute tracheal collapse and postoperative hypocalcaemia. Discussion of hypocalcaemia is inappropriate in this question; hypoparathyroidism will occur only if all the parathyroids are removed, which will not happen in a subtotal thyroidectomy. Although tracheal collapse, classically, is a rare complication after resection of extensive malignancy, it can occur after subtotal resection of a large goitre.

CHAPTER 6

Specialized general anaesthesia

6-1 Write an essay on the anaesthetist and maternal mortality.

OUTLINE PLAN

Triennial reports

mechanism

Common causes of death

discuss figures over the years

Anaesthetic factors

general anaesthesia

conduction anaesthesia

hypovolaemia

Difficult intubation

Aspiration

Compare conduction and general anaesthesia

Current suggestions

The examiners are giving candidates free rein: you can choose what emphasis to give your answer, and there are many satisfactory approaches. There are some things that must, however, be mentioned whatever your approach, and these are: to define what is meant by maternal mortality; to mention the triennial reports; to discuss aspiration of gastric contents; and to discuss the pros and cons of general anaesthesia and epidural anaesthesia for Caesarean section. Other topics, though important in a comprehensive article on the subject, may be necessary in your answer only if they fit well with your approach, for example the details of failed intubation drill or precise figures from triennial reports.

Possible opening sentences:

Anaesthesia continues to be one of the main causes of death associated with childbirth.

The results of confidential enquiries into maternal deaths in England and Wales are published by the Department of Health at three-yearly intervals.

A maternal death is the death of a woman while pregnant or within

42 days of the termination of pregnancy from all causes except those caused by coincidental accidents.

Anaesthetic deaths come under two headings: those caused by anaesthesia itself and those in which anaesthesia contributed to the problem that resulted directly in the death.

The first sentence is too self-evident. The second and third are good. The fourth would be better later, when describing the form of the triennial reports.

Note that the definition of a maternal death is a somewhat shortened version of the official definition.

Triennial reports
mechanism

Common causes of death
hypertensive disease
pulmonary embolism
hypovolaemia
anaesthesia
discuss figures over the years

Discuss these generally in relation to one another unless you *know* the current position of anaesthesia in the *latest* triennial report. Now move away from general discussion to the anaesthetic factors.

Anaesthetic factors
general anaesthesia
   difficult intubation
   aspiration of gastric contents
conduction anaesthesia
   overdose
hypovolaemia
pre-eclampsia

Some would discuss aspiration before difficult intubation as being the most common *direct* factor, but in practice aspiration is unusual if there are not problems with intubation as well. All items in the list require considerable detail.

Pre-eclampsia will need to be mentioned at a number of points in the essay.

Difficult intubation
causes
action

Aspiration
causes

prophylaxis
treatment

Conduction anaesthesia

At the time of writing, it seems that epidural anaesthesia is safer for Caesarean section in that the number of deaths due to anaesthesia has fallen in the league table as the relative number of epidurals has increased. This does not *prove* that the one is due to the other; it could be that monitoring and staffing have improved at the same time. You must know the current stage of this discussion for your answer.

pros and cons of GA
   precautions
      against overdose
      against hypotension

Hypovolaemia

recognition
action

Remember that an epidural does not guarantee aspiration will not occur: a profoundly hypotensive woman lying on her back may be confused and have obtunded reflexes.

Obstetric anaesthesia is the subject of frequent pronouncements and recommendations. Read relevant editorials so that you know what is topical.

Current suggestions

adequate preoperative assessment
prefer epidural (spinal)
staffing

Staffing refers to the resident anaesthetist, experienced back-up, and suitable assistance.

6-2   Discuss the anaesthetic considerations of pre-eclampsia.

OUTLINE PLAN

Mild

Lumbar epidural

for labour and vaginal delivery
check for contraindications
advantages
discuss treatment of hypotension

Severe: define

Physiological disturbances

Drug treatment

antihypertensive

anticonvulsant

Anaesthetic technique

general anaesthesia

special difficulties

monitoring

chosen technique

In high dependency

monitor: especially fluids

There are two approaches to the opening sentence: either a definition of pre-eclampsia (you will need to give one at some stage), or a summary of the main anaesthetic difficulties.

Pre-eclampsia is characterized by the triad of hypertension, proteinuria and oedema, and is defined as severe when specific signs are present.

The main difficulties faced by the anaesthetist asked to attend a woman with pre-eclampsia are difficult venous access, oedema of the airway, a tendency to sudden severe hypertension, the likelihood of fitting, and clotting abnormalities.

Pre-eclampsia is still an important cause of maternal mortality, and the anaesthetist has an important role to play in reducing the risk to the mother and the fetus.

The third sentence is poor for three reasons. First, it is stating the obvious. Secondly, it is not strictly correct, because pre-eclampsia is only an expression of the underlying condition, which is hypertensive disease of pregnancy. Thirdly, although this is not the sort of detail that examiners will *expect* from candidates under the stress of examination, writing of anaesthetists 'having a role to play' is a long-winded and metaphorical way (the metaphor being of an actor on the stage) of writing that 'the anaesthetist can reduce the risk...'. In examination essays, as in most other forms of writing, fewer words are better. Examiners are not fooled by padding.

The answer is best considered in two parts: mild and severe pre-eclampsia.

Mild

Lumbar epidural

for labour and vaginal delivery

first check:

routine contraindications

clotting

circulating volume
advantages of epidural
   reduction of maternal stress
   helps control blood pressure
   helps improve placental circulation?
   allows operative delivery
discuss treatment of hypotension

There is no need for details of placement of the epidural, but clear details and figures are needed for clotting tests. There can be a fine balance between hypotension caused by the epidural and hypertension caused by attempts to correct the hypotension; this needs a well-thought out scheme.

Severe: define

Physiological disturbances

   investigations

The question asks for 'anaesthetic considerations', which, for severe pre-eclampsia, implies urgent delivery by Caesarean section. You should not discuss prolonged holding treatment on the ward — that is an obstetric consideration.

Drug treatment

   antihypertensive
   anticonvulsant

Anaesthetic technique

   paediatrician*
   (epidural)
   (spinal)
   general anaesthesia
     how differs from standard
       difficult intubation
       hypertension on intubation
       difficulties with circulating volume
     monitoring
     chosen induction technique
     maintenance

'Paediatrician' has an asterisk because it is a good idea to make more than usually certain that the paediatrician will be present. Although the prime concern of the anaesthetist is the mother, sometimes there is no one else there with the skill to resuscitate a 'flat' baby. The anaesthetist will not be able to leave a pre-eclamptic mother at all.

The brackets indicate that regional techniques are not ruled out but discussion of them must be circumspect. It is more likely that you would give a general anaesthetic.

There is nothing special about reversal or postoperative pain relief, but you must mention that the risk of fitting remains, though declining, for 24 hours at least.

In high dependency

monitor: especially fluids

6-3 <u>**How may the anaesthetist influence intracranial pressure in a patient presenting for craniotomy with a space-occupying lesion?**</u>

OUTLINE PLAN

Volume/pressure diagram

Altering cerebral blood flow

carbon dioxide tension
arterial blood pressure
   autoregulation
   cerebral perfusion pressure
   hypotension
anaesthetic techniques and drugs

Avoiding cerebral venous congestion

position
ventilation
maintain relaxation

Reducing volume of brain tissue

diuresis
steroids

Reducing CSF volume

spinal drainage

The first half of this answer will be a description of the physiology of intracranial pressure.

Opening sentences:

> The intracranial contents are brain tissue, cerebrospinal fluid (CSF) and blood, and it is by indirectly altering the amount of blood that the anaesthetist has most effect.

> The skull will allow some increase of its contents without harm, but once the intracranial pressure (ICP) starts to increase, it increases rapidly.

All that is needed in the opening sentence is a lead-in to the physiology, and a sketched graph of intracranial pressure against volume should appear in your answer.

The abbreviations CSF and ICP can be used if identified, but do not use any others, for instance CBF for cerebral blood flow, CBV for cerebral blood volume, CPP for cerebral perfusion pressure. These abbreviations are too similar, especially with some people's handwriting, and can make reading of the answer difficult.

Volume and pressure
  diagram

Altering cerebral blood volume: cerebral blood flow
  carbon dioxide tension
    detail
  arterial blood pressure
    autoregulation
    cerebral perfusion pressure
      intubation
      skin incision
    hypotension
      intentional
      unintentional
  anaesthetic techniques and drugs
    inhalational agents
    (cerebral metabolic rate)
    anticonvulsants
      postoperative pain relief

Beware of detailed descriptions of complicated studies of the effects of various agents on cerebral metabolic rate. If drugs are used sensibly, they do not have any practical effect on intracranial pressure, and certainly not if compared with the effect of $PaCO_2$.

Altering cerebral blood volume: venous congestion
  position: of body
    of neck
  ventilation
  maintain relaxation

Reducing volume of brain tissue
  diuresis
  steroids

Reducing CSF volume
  spinal drainage

Do not discuss treatment of raised intracranial pressure on the intensive care unit or the insertion of bolts for monitoring. The question is about a patient 'presenting for craniotomy', and the main concern of the anaesthetist is to prevent rises in intracranial pressure before the skull is opened.

6-4 Discuss the management of general anaesthesia for a 4 kg infant who requires a pyloromyotomy (Ramstedt's operation).

OUTLINE PLAN

Preoperative assessment

history
physical examination
expected biochemical picture

Preoperative management

nasogastric tube
intravenous infusion
correct deficit
maintenance
objectives

Operative management

premedication
induction
awake intubation?
maintenance
drugs, equipment, fluids, monitoring
reversal
postoperative fluids & analgesia

Possible opening sentences:

Congential hypertrophic pyloric stenosis is a condition occurring more commonly in first-born male infants, in which obstruction of the pylorus causes persistent vomiting.

Surgery for pyloric stenosis should be delayed until the biochemical disturbance, classically a hypochloraemic alkalosis, has been treated.

The main problems of congenital pyloric stenosis for the anaesthetist are the biochemical disturbances and the risks of induction of anaesthesia in a patient with a full stomach.

The first sentence is true, but is a surgical not an anaesthetic introduction. Either of the other two sentences is good and will lead into the first topic of the answer: the preoperative management. In most hospitals, the paediatricians will be responsible for this, but your answer must include some details about this phase of the treatment as it is important in the assessment of whether the infant is fit for anaesthesia. Do not include large amounts of detail of preoperative management at the expense of detail of the anaesthetic procedure.

Preoperative assessment

history

physical examination
expected biochemical picture
explanation from physiology
assessment of severity

You need only discuss history and examination relevant to the assessment of the infant as being fit for operation. Do not be sidetracked into considering other diseases or writing 'if otherwise fit' or similar phrases. The question specifies 4 kg, so this child *is* otherwise fit.

Preoperative management

not urgent surgery: 12–72 hours
nasogastric tube
intravenous infusion
   correct deficit
      2:1 5% dextrose:0.9% saline at 50–150 ml/kg
      (mmol Na = deficit × body weight × 0.6)
   maintenance
      4% dextrose/0.18% saline at 4 ml/kg/h
      3 mmol KCl/kg/day when satisfactory urine output
objectives
   serum Cl > 90, Na > 135, HCO_3 < 24 mmol/L

You should not be learning facts from this book. The figures given here, although satisfactory, are given because you will be expected to give some. If yours differ from ours, go and read about the subject. Note that in your *plan* you are likely to jot down a formula that you have learned — but the question specifies the weight of the child and you can give absolute values.

Operative management

premedication: atropine
induction: aspirate NG, rapid sequence
   drugs
   ET tube
   awake intubation?
maintenance
   drugs
   equipment
   fluids
   monitoring
      NB temperature
reversal
postoperatively
   fluids
   analgesia

At the stage of Part 1 FCAnaes, you would not be expected to give this anaesthetic unsupervised, so this is an unlikely question. The candidate for Part 3 must be able to discuss topics such as: should you give opioids? is an inhalational induction a possibility?

6-5 Discuss the anaesthetic management of a 2-year-old child undergoing a course of radiotherapy.

OUTLINE PLAN

General problems

patient isolated

monitoring

minimize disruption of normal life

emotional problems

medical problems

Anaesthetic management

premedication

Standard general anaesthesia

induction

intravenous, inhalational

maintenance

Ketamine

advantages

disadvantages

Monitoring

television

telemetry

Opening sentences:

> Radiotherapy is used in the management of a variety of malignant diseases in childhood including acute leukaemia, Wilms' tumour, retinoblastoma and central nervous system tumours.

> Courses of radiotherapy require children to lie alone and absolutely still for short periods, and the treatment may need to be repeated daily.

There is nothing wrong with the first sentence, but the second one gets to the point better and is a good introduction to a general discussion of the problems before you reach the specific points of anaesthetic management.

There is no need for any discussion of different radiotherapeutic procedures (marking up, treatments, scanning, different machines) because they have no bearing on the anaesthetic technique.

General problems
    repeated sedation or general anaesthesia
    patient isolated, but need rapid access
    monitoring difficulties
    minimize disruption of normal life
        rapid recovery
    emotional problems
        child and parents
    medical problems
        nausea and vomiting
        bone marrow failure
        cardiomyopathy
        radiation pneumonitis
        of specific conditions

There is no need for an exhaustive list of medical complications in children with malignant disease. Give a general list and a few illustrative problems.

Anaesthetic management
    premedication
    involve parents

An older child may need to be involved in discussions about premedication (although once old enough to take part in these discussions they may also be old enough to tolerate radiotherapy without anaesthesia). A child of two is not old enough, and writing 'Premedication should be discussed with the parents and patient' shows you are not thinking clearly about the subject.

If the child will not lie still, then full general anaesthesia is required; there is no place for sedation techniques. The choice is between standard general anaesthesia and ketamine, and the advantages and disadvantages must be discussed.

Standard general anaesthesia
    secure long-term venous access
    induction
        intravenous, inhalational
    maintenance

Discuss these topics relating specifically to the question. Children rapidly get used to the idea of 'magic cream and a pinprick' or breathing themselves asleep, or else they rapidly become unmanageable. Repeated induction is a different problem from induction on a single occasion; that is one of the reasons the question has been asked, and you must show the examiners that you realize that.

You need to discuss details of maintenance, which is likely to depend on personal preference as much as anything. Radiotherapy is a regional specialty and not every anaesthetist, even at Part 3 FCAnaes, will have been faced with the problem of giving anaesthetics for repeated procedures. The problems are similar in, for instance, burns units, but if you are using that experience on which to base this answer remember that radiotherapy is painless.

If you have given this type of anaesthetic, write 'In our unit the preferred technique...' and give the reasons for the preference. Otherwise, anyone taking Part 3 should be able to discuss in general terms the advantages and disadvantages of face mask, laryngeal mask, and endotracheal tube; spontaneous and controlled ventilation; choice of inhalational agent, or of intravenous agent: *for this circumstance.*

Ketamine is worth discussing entirely separately:

Ketamine
  advantages
    intramuscular injection (?)
    cardiovascular stability
    ventilation well maintained
    airway reflexes relatively preserved
  disadvantages
    repeated intramuscular injection
    salivation
    airway not guaranteed
    purposeless movements
    prolonged recovery
      sleep and eating problems

Discussion of ketamine produces a reflex statement about emergence phenomena, of little relevance in a 2-year-old.

Monitoring
  television
  telemetry
  ability to stop treatment

Television allows a close view of the patient; telemetry allows monitored variables to be transmitted without wires to equipment outside the treatment room. Which variables should be monitored is not a topic that should need any prompting in this book.

6-6 Discuss the perioperative management of a 29-week premature neonate with a congenital diaphragmatic hernia.

OUTLINE PLAN

Problems of neonatal physiology
  respiratory

    compliance
    vascular resistance
    apnoeic episodes
    temperature control

Problems of neonatal anaesthesia

    size
    oxygenation
    fluids

Preoperatively

    NG tube
    oxygen and ventilation
    fluids
    transport to theatre

In operating theatre

    check lines
    induction
        monitoring
    maintenance
        heat loss
        monitoring
            oximetry
            airway pressure
            blood loss

Postoperatively

    gastric suction and IV fluids
    indications for extubation
    indications for continued ventilation

This is a Part 3 FCAnaes question and few anaesthetists sitting the examination will have seen the condition. If you are writing this question from the textbooks, say so in your answer. The same is true if asked the question in a viva. If you have never seen a case, you are unlikely to be able to give as good an answer as someone who has, but what is important is to show you know what the problems are, rather than showing an ability to solve them.

Remember that much of the question and therefore many of the marks hang on the problems of dealing with premature infants. An answer that is perfect on every detail of the anatomy, surgery and best anaesthetic technique for all the different grades of diaphragmatic hernia will not gain the pass mark if it contains nothing about, for instance, prevention of hypothermia.

A fairly general, non-committal opening sentence is probably best:

Congenital diaphragmatic hernia is a rare condition in which the main anaesthetic problems are related to difficulties in ventilation and oxygenation.

A *brief* summary of presentation, diagnosis and investigations could be included in the opening paragraph. It is worth mentioning that the condition may be associated with other abnormalities, such as congenital heart disease, but further details are not necessary. Do not use the abbreviation CDH, which is more familiar for congenital dislocation of the hip. Once you have established that you are describing congenital diaphragmatic hernia, you can shorten it: 'Congenital diaphragmatic hernia is usually on the left side . . . and the prognosis depends on the degree of pulmonary hypoplasia caused by the hernia'; or refer to it as 'the condition' or other suitable expression.

Problems of neonatal physiology

respiratory
> low pulmonary compliance (pneumothorax)
> increased pulmonary vascular resistance
> apnoeic episodes

temperature control
haemostasis
glucose metabolism

Problems of neonatal anaesthesia

size: 1–2 kg
> venous access
> intubation

oxygenation
> hypoxia and hyperoxia (retrolental fibroplasia)

fluids

In your full answer, there can be considerable overlap between the lists under the two headings, particularly when discussing the respiratory system. The advantage of dealing first with general neonatal problems is that you cannot then overlook them, and you can also concentrate better on the specific problems of the condition without being distracted. For instance, if you deal once with temperature control and suggest an ideal ambient temperature, then there is no need to keep repeating 'preoperatively the temperature must be maintained . . .', 'the transport incubator must be at 34°C . . .', 'the operating theatre must be kept warm . . .', and so on.

Preoperatively

nursed semi-upright
NG tube
humidified oxygen
> ventilate if necessary

fluids

check biochemistry
transport to theatre
In operating theatre
check lines
induction
　avoid nitrous oxide & mask ventilation
　monitoring

Intravenous infusions and arterial lines commonly become blocked or disconnected when patients are transferred around hospitals; mentioning such points shows that you can think practically, not just theoretically.

maintenance
　drugs
　technique
　heat loss
　monitoring
　　especially
　　　oximetry
　　　airway pressure (pneumothorax)
　　　blood loss

Good points for discussion are the use of opioids and whether hand or machine is better for ventilation.

Although temperature control was dealt with in the earlier list, specific details of how you use cotton wool, aluminized blankets and a heating mattress fit well here.

Postoperatively
gastric suction and IV fluids
indications for extubation
indications for continued ventilation
　perhaps pulmonary vasodilator
　extracorporeal membrane oxygenation

This is a question about perioperative management not paediatric intensive care. Details are not needed of extreme treatments for continuing grave hypoxia but these topics do provide a way of rounding off the answer.

6-7　What are the anaesthetic considerations of hip replacement surgery? What are the relative merits of the various techniques of anaesthesia?

OUTLINE PLAN

Problems from patient
old age

    arthritis
      other joints
        intubation
    rheumatoid arthritis
      systemic effects
      drug therapy

Problems from operation

    access
    prosthesis
    blood loss

Postoperative considerations

    thromboembolism

Regional techniques versus general anaesthesia

    brief descriptions
    advantages and disadvantages
      relate to problems

Although there seem to be two parts to this question, it is really asking you simply to write an essay about anaesthesia for hip surgery. A number of things should come to mind immediately: elderly patients, other diseases, other joints, cement, regional versus general. These topics are the main points for discussion. Your opening sentence should pick up on one or more of these.

> Most patients who present for this procedure are elderly and suffering from osteoarthritis or rheumatoid arthritis.

> The main anaesthetic decision for this operation is whether to give a general anaesthetic, a regional technique, or to combine them.

The first sentence starts well, but the statement of orthopaedic diagnoses has little impact. It is a better opener than the second sentence, which is moving too soon onto the second part of the question, but it is improved by expanding the problems of the elderly patients who present for this operation.

> Most patients who present for this procedure are elderly and have intercurrent conditions simply because of age or as a complication of their orthopaedic diagnosis, an important one of which, rheumatoid arthritis, is a general disorder of connective tissues.

Your plan now starts with the expected problems. Do not leap in with discussions of difficult intubation; general considerations come before specific ones.

Problems from patient

old age
arthritis
   other peripheral joints
     position on table
   neck and jaw
     intubation

There are many questions in which age is a factor (see prostatectomy, p. 123). You should prepare a standard paragraph that you can insert in appropriate essays, giving the likely conditions and the preoperative investigations dictated by them. There is no need for specific details of *how* you would treat intercurrent disease, but you must write that treatment may be necessary.

A *short* discussion of approaches to difficult intubation can lead to the next section, on the problems of rheumatoid arthritis. Do not forget to mention, in your enthusiasm at having remembered all the problems of the elderly patient, that young patients who have severely diseased rheumatoid joints often have many of the other manifestations of the condition.

rheumatoid arthritis
   cardiopulmonary dysfunction
   haematology
   drug therapy
   venous access

Problems from operation

access to patient on table
bone cement and air embolus
blood loss

Postoperative considerations

thromboembolism

Now you have dealt with the most important problems of hip surgery, you can discuss the anaesthetic technique by referring to them. As mentioned earlier, the 'various techniques' is really asking for a discussion of regional versus general; it is not asking for a full description of anaesthetic techniques, from the drugs used for premedication to drugs for reversal. Even less are the examiners asking for the knee-jerk response, 'First I would go to the ward to see the patient . . .,' that many candidates — incorrectly — believe has to preface any discussion of anaesthesia.

Regional techniques

brief description
advantages and disadvantages

General anaesthesia
brief description
advantages and disadvantages

Combination techniques

At Part 1, simple statements of a regional and a general technique are enough; in fact, the wording of this question is much more suitable for Part 3, because the 'relative merits' of techniques are not what anaesthetists learn in their first year or so of anaesthetic practice. A candidate for Part 3 must be aware of the current thinking in a number of debates in the specialty, and regional versus general for hip surgery, particularly for fractured neck of femur, is a long-running one. Opinions change. At the time of writing it is believed that regional anaesthesia has a better immediate outcome but that the more long-term outcome is the same as for general. The same is true for blood loss: that deliberate hypotension reduces perioperative loss but not overall loss. These are not cast-iron facts; later, larger, better controlled studies may alter our ideas. Candidates for Part 3 must be up-to-date.

6-8 Describe the anaesthetic management of a previously healthy young adult who requires thoracotomy following a stab wound in the chest.

OUTLINE PLAN

Main complications
haemothorax
pneumothorax
cardiac tamponade

Injuries to
great vessels
large airways
oesophagus
lung

Preoperative assessment and management
history
airway
breathing
circulation
palpate for surgical emphysema and crepitus
action (with appropriate urgency)
   chest drain

Induction of anaesthesia
monitoring
choice of tracheal tube

Position for surgery

Maintenance

Ventilation

one-lung anaesthesia
underwater seal drains

Surgical problems

Recovery phase

extubation?
pain relief
bronchopleural fistula

Start with a straightforward statement of the main complications of this injury.

The three most important complications of this injury are haemothorax, pneumothorax and cardiac tamponade.

Another possible way to open is to stress the importance of careful assessment.

Fit, young adults can appear well despite serious injury and the rapidity with which their condition can worsen means that assessment must be rapid yet thorough.

Both these approaches can be combined in the opening paragraph. Before describing your method of assessment, describe the consequences of the main complications and briefly describe the other structures at risk.

Main complications

haemothorax
pneumothorax
   tension
cardiac tamponade
immediate management (here or below)

Injuries to

great vessels
large airways
oesophagus
lung

You may prefer to leave all of management until later; or you may choose to write a sentence or two early in your answer about how, for example, to manage an obvious and obviously life-threatening pneumothorax.

Preoperative assessment and management

history
airway
breathing

circulation
   is it blood loss or tamponade?
   circulatory access
palpate for surgical emphysema and crepitus
investigations
action (with appropriate urgency)
   chest drain

'History' includes the site of the injury, the type of knife and whether it is still in the patient. Where you will site chest drains and venous lines depends also on the site of injury; give some examples of possible difficulties.

Induction of anaesthesia

monitoring
check all lines and drains
drugs
rapid sequence induction
   choice of tracheal tube

Position for surgery

check tracheal tube

Maintenance

maintain saturation
nitrous oxide?
profound hypotension
fluid management

These patients can require massive transfusion, and some detail is needed on how you match the type of fluid to estimated blood loss. Do not forget urine output as a guide to the management of fluids.

Ventilation

one-lung anaesthesia
re-expansion
underwater seal drains

Surgical problems

The discussion of one-lung anaesthesia does not need to be as detailed as in the question about pneumonectomy for carcinoma (see opposite); this patient is previously fit and healthy. However, you can include more detail about chest drains in this answer.

These explorations can be difficult surgically, especially if the oesophagus needs repair or even more if damage to major vessels or the heart means that cardiopulmonary bypass is required. These possible difficulties should be mentioned, but no detail is required.

Recovery phase

extubation?

pain relief
complications
bronchopleural fistula

An early bronchopleural fistula is more likely than after routine pneumonectomy. Include a brief discussion of how you manage one.

6-9 Discuss the anaesthetic management of a patient who requires right pneumonectomy for bronchial carcinoma.

OUTLINE PLAN

Respiratory

investigations
effect on operative risk

Cardiovascular

ischaemic heart disease
right ventricular function

Other systems

endocrine disturbances
Eaton–Lambert

Preoperative preparation

treat infection and bronchospasm

Anaesthetic technique

drugs and monitoring

One-lung anaesthesia

physiology
double-lumen tracheal tubes
my choice
hypoxia

Postoperative management

respiratory
analgesia
complications
broncho-pleural fistula

There are two contrasting dangers in this question, which is firmly of Part 3 standard rather than Part 1. The first danger is concentrating too soon on the intraoperative problems of pneumonectomy and one-lung ventilation. The second danger is that of spending too long writing about the medical complications of bronchial carcinoma, which are many and can affect the anaesthetic management. As when answering any clinical question: *common things occur commonly*. Every patient who has a pneumonectomy has to be ventilated on one lung but only a few will have Eaton-Lambert syndrome. Deal with the question as you would deal with the patient, by keeping the problems of one-lung ventilation foremost, but maintaining an index of suspicion about the rarer complications. The opening sentence is a good opportunity to show the examiner that your priorities are correct.

> This operation poses the anaesthetist the practical difficulties of maintaining ventilation via one, perhaps diseased, lung, in a patient who often has concurrent smoking-related disease and who uncommonly may have non-metastatic complications of the carcinoma.

This is a long and somewhat awkward first sentence that may be better as two, but which gives a firm outline to the answer. It is a large topic and there is no time for waffle, so get straight on to the preoperative assessment.

Respiratory
> history, examination
>> investigations
>>> effect on operative risk

You are not asked how to diagnose bronchial carcinoma. As an anaesthetist on a preoperative visit, you would not enquire about a history of exposure to asbestos nor look for signs of clubbing. You would want to know about dyspnoea, wheeze and sputum production. Keep your answer relevant to the question as asked.

Do not simply give a list of all possible investigations. Some patients with operable lung cancer have no functional respiratory symptoms — they may have had just a single episode of haemoptysis — and there is then no need to know the arterial blood gas tensions. Explain to the examiner which investigations you would want, in what sort of patients, and explain also the significance of abnormalities.

Cardiovascular
> ischaemic heart disease
> right ventricular function
> history and examination
> investigations (CXR here)

Beware of statements such as, 'All patients with lung cancer are likely to have ischaemic heart disease . . .' : 10% of patients with lung cancer have never smoked. Although a chest X-ray can be counted as an investigation of the respiratory system, it may be better dealt with in this section when both relevant systems have been discussed.

Other systems
> endocrine disturbances

investigations
metastatic disease
Eaton–Lambert

These need a separate paragraph, giving the anaesthetist's view, not the physician's. You must deal with the myasthenic syndrome, either here or later when discussing drugs used during anaesthesia.

Preoperative preparation

stop smoking
treat infection and bronchospasm
ventilatory 'exercises'
   physiotherapy

Anaesthetic technique

premedication
induction, routine maintenance
monitoring

Some anaesthetists always use invasive monitoring of blood pressure; others just use a cuff. Beware of statements that 'The anaesthetist must . . .'. If you like always to use an arterial cannula and an internal jugular cannula, give the examiner your reasons.

One-lung anaesthesia

physiology
   dependent and non-dependent; ventilation/perfusion
double-lumen tracheal tubes
   my choice
      confirmation of position
maintenance of anaesthesia
avoidance and treatment of hypoxia

The physiology of one-lung anaesthesia is an important part of this question.

You do not need to give a detailed description of all the available double-lumen tubes; describe the one you are most familiar with and your technique of ensuring and securing placement. When you discuss the general difference between left and right-sided tubes, remember that this question specifies *right pneumonectomy*.

There is no *necessity* for a double-lumen tube; the lung to be excised can be packed away by the surgeon and the open bronchial stump can be sutured closed quickly enough to ensure that no harm will come to the patient.

Postoperative management

respiratory
analgesia

complications
    bleeding and hypotension
    pericardial herniation
    arrhythmias
    broncho-pleural fistula

The anaesthetic management includes a brief description of broncho-pleural fistula and its recognition in the recovery room, but not a detailed description of the management of a chronic fistula.

6-10 Discuss the possible complications of general anaesthesia for adults in the dental chair.

OUTLINE PLAN

Assessment — suitable?

Equipment
    especially chair to go flat

Induction

Maintenance
    pack and nasal mask

Initial problems with the airway
    obstruction
        causes
    apnoea

Complicated problems with the airway
    risk of aspiration

Cardiovascular complications
    the 'single operator'
    should all be flat?
    hypotension
    arrhythmias

Problems in recovery

Not a trick question, but there are two easy traps. We are more used to thinking about children for anaesthesia in the dental chair; and for adults we tend to use sedation techniques. This question is explicit; it is about general anaesthesia for adults and you must stick to the question asked.

Opening sentences:

The standard anaesthetic technique for adults in the dental chair is an intravenous induction followed by oxygen, nitrous oxide and a volatile agent, breathed spontaneously by nasal mask.

Anaesthesia in the dental chair implies short procedures done as day-case surgery in a dental surgery or clinic, and in adults is likely to be necessary only for the otherwise fit but very anxious or mentally sub-normal.

Either of these sentences sets the scene and helps to define the limits of your answer to the examiner: intubation is not included; there will be no discussion of ventilators; you will not be going to see the patient on the ward preoperatively; assessment does not include laboratory investigations.

Having avoided the traps of children and sedation, you must now obey the golden rule of answering examination questions: *be relevant*. There are no complications of general anaesthesia under these circumstances that *cannot* happen in any anaesthetic, so you must be selective and discuss those of special relevance to the situation presented to you. Sit for a moment and imagine: an anxious patient, for a short procedure, with a standard anaesthetic technique, a shared airway, and the dental chair. What are the most likely things to go wrong? There are only two important headings: airway (though there is a list of sub-headings) and syncope.

Now start the plan with your chosen anaesthetic technique for the uncomplicated case.

Assessment — suitable?

Equipment
for emergency: tubes, resuscitation
    especially chair to go flat
monitoring

Induction

Maintenance
agent
nasal mask
pack

You need a full description of your chosen technique, and a reason for your choice of drugs. There is no need to describe your check procedures in detail, but you must know how to get the chair flat quickly, and suction is also worth a special mention.

Initial problems with the airway
obstruction
cause
    pack
    blocked nose
    loss of tone
    laryngospasm

apnoea
(bronchospasm)

For each of these, you need to say how you diagnose it, why it occurs, and how you would deal with it. Bronchospasm is in brackets because it only needs a brief mention; it is unlikely (asthmatics should not be treated as day cases) but dangerous if unrecognized.

Complicated problems with the airway

vomiting
regurgitation

A patient sitting in a dental chair cannot regurgitate, though may do so when laid down at the end of the procedure.

Cardiovascular complications

the 'single operator'
should all be flat?
hypotension
  with normal heart rate
  with bradycardia
arrhythmias

The very rare, unexpected ventricular fibrillation aside, it is hypotension that damages people in the dental chair. This is a good point in the essay to discuss the inadvisability for dentists to be their own anaesthetist and to raise the question whether there is ever a need to operate with the patient sitting. These details are for Part 3. Candidates for Part 1 should be able to discuss the other headings, and the appropriate management.

Problems in recovery

staffing and equipment

The problems of recovery are no different from those that occur elsewhere, but when operations are short and there may be a large number of patients dealt with in a short time, it is much easier for patients to be overlooked.

6-11 Write short notes on general anaesthesia for laser surgery of the larynx.

OUTLINE PLAN

Surgical advantages

Specific disadvantages

Specific anaesthetic approach

tracheal tubes

smoke inhalation

airway fire

General problems of laryngeal surgery

primary airway difficulties

competition for airway

circulatory disturbances

Preoperative visit

general condition

airway

Anaesthetic technique

principles

especially oxygenation and ventilation

Surgical advances sometimes cause anaesthetic difficulties. (Other recent techniques include laparoscopic cholecystectomy and lithotriptic techniques. Any advance that has been the subject of editorials or reviews in the anaesthetic journals is a fair question in an examination, though usually this type of advance is for Part 3 rather than Part 1.) The examiners will not expect candidates to be familiar with all new techniques; not all hospitals have the equipment. Questions on new techniques can be a gift for those candidates who are familiar with a technique, while those who have never seen it may feel discriminated against. However, Part 3 is an examination not just of what you have seen but also of what you have read, and there is more to laryngeal surgery than knowing about lasers. Candidates familiar with laser surgery may be in danger of failing the question if they ignore the more general considerations.

Short notes is not a licence to dispense with a logical plan, nor to cover the page in ill-organized lists of abbreviations.

An opening summary sentence, or summary list, is still worthwhile.

> Laryngeal surgery using a laser enables effective surgery of sometimes difficult lesions, but in addition to the usual problems of the shared airway there are the unusual dangers of damage to operating theatre staff and of fires in the airway.

There is no need to describe how lasers work. Start the question with the specific problems of laser surgery. Although this is the reverse of the more usual approach to an answer, it enables a less repetitive answer and draws the examiner's attention to your understanding of the difficulties.

Surgical advantages

Specific disadvantages

to staff

of fire

Specific anaesthetic approach

tracheal tubes

volatile agents/intravenous infusion

may need to deal with

smoke inhalation

airway fire

General problems of laryngeal surgery

patency of airway

difficult intubation

competition for airway

circulatory disturbances

The special difficulties dealt with, you can now concentrate on anaesthesia for laryngeal surgery, using the standard approach starting with preoperative assessment.

Preoperative visit

general condition

airway

premedication

Anaesthetic technique

principles of anaesthetic approach

The surgeon wants a good view of immobile vocal cords, and the anaesthetist wants a rapid recovery of the protective reflexes: easier to write than to achieve.

induction

maintenance

drugs

oxygenation and ventilation

monitoring

recovery

Lists earlier in the answer included tracheal tubes and possibly some of the drugs. The various techniques of maintaining gas exchange may be better in this more general section of the answer. There is a conflict between wanting to supply a high oxygen concentration for the patient and not wanting to encourage conflagration. This is a topic not well suited to short notes because it requires discussion, but just because the examiners have specified short notes does not prevent your writing a paragraph of discussion if you wish.

6-12 Write short notes on: a) complications of neurolytic block; b) neurolytic agents; c) transcutaneous nerve stimulation (TENS); d) cryo-analgesia.

OUTLINE PLAN

Complications of neurolytic block

> related to site of injection
> remote (e.g. sphincter)
> late (denervation)
> avoidance

Neurolytic agents

> drugs
> draw up table for comparisons

TENS

> description
>> mechanics
>> physiology
> uses
> advantages and disadvantages

Cryo-analgesia

> description
>> mechanics
>> physiology
> uses
> adverse effects

Short notes does not mean an unconnected list of isolated facts, with undefined abbreviations scattered here and there: work from a plan as with any other answer. You cannot expect to pass a short notes question if you fail to answer *any one part* satisfactorily.

There is no need for an opening sentence.

Complications of neurolytic block

> failure of block
> intravascular injection
> spread to other structures, e.g. spinal cord
> sphincter disturbance
> complications of denervation
>> sloughing, neuritis, anaesthesia dolorosa
>> corneal damage
> how to avoid (brief)

The easiest way to answer the next section is with a quick (but neat) comparative table.

Neurolytic agents

phenol, alcohol, chlorocresol
compare for: concentration, baricity, pain on injection,
    onset, spread, local analgesia effect, differential block,
        toxicity, propensity for chemical neuritis, uses

The examiners have defined the abbreviation TENS, so you do not need to.

TENS

description
    portable electrical stimulator
    patient adjusts
    endogenous opioids, substantia gelatinosa
    placebo?
uses
    localized mild to moderate pain
        postherpetic, phantom limb, causalgia, low
        back pain
advantages: no serious disadvantages, non-invasive
disadvantages: skin reactions, non-responders

Cryo-analgesia

description
    of the machinery
    of the neural effect
uses
    atypical facial pain
    intercostal neuralgia
    post-thoracotomy
adverse effects
    neuritis
    soreness at site of insertion of probe

Each line in these lists should be expanded to a sentence or two. Although we wrote that you must write on all four parts of the question, that does not mean you must be able to write in equal detail on all topics in the lists. For example, we have listed atypical facial pain, intercostal neuralgia and pain after thoracotomy as examples for the use of cryo-analgesia. You may have seen other uses; you may know about atypical facial pain in some detail but know little about pain after thoracotomy. Choose your examples from those you know; there is nothing wrong with then adding a summary statement, 'This technique is also useful in . . .'.

CHAPTER 7

Intensive care

7-1   What forms of ventilatory support are used for patients undergoing mechanical ventilation?

OUTLINE PLAN

Full ventilation

   patient-initiated

Partial support

   intermittent breaths
   preset volume
   assist

Negative pressure ventilation

   iron lung, cuirass, rocking bed

For each describe: for — against — uses

Other forms of ventilation

   high frequency
   variations of intra-cycle pressure and flow

This is not an easy question. Ventilatory support is to some extent a matter of fashion, and the journals covering intensive care are full of abbreviations and acronyms for all manner of novel ways of avoiding delivering a straightforward tidal volume a set number of times per minute. The same method of support might have a number of abbreviations associated with it, originating from the manufacturers of the available ventilators. Because of this, rather than trying to think of all possible modes of ventilation and describing them in turn, it is better to deal with them by principle. Although it is not necessary in the answer, you could start your plan simply by jotting down as many abbreviations as you can think of. Grouping them and underlining those in common use lead you to a structured answer.

Another reason for difficulty is that the question asks for 'ventilatory support': does this include positive end-expiratory pressure (PEEP) and continuous end-expiratory pressure (CPAP)? These techniques aid oxygenation, which can prevent the hypoxia that makes it difficult to settle some patients, but they are not supporting the ventilation — the movement of air in and out of the lungs — directly. Sometimes when answering a question you have to define to the examiner how you have interpreted the question and you can do this in your opening sentence or paragraph.

Opening sentences:

> Most of the specialized modes of ventilation have been introduced either to make it easier to settle patients on ventilators or to make it easier to wean the patients from them.

> Patients requiring mechanical ventilation can be given a predetermined tidal volume a set number of times per minute, as in the operating theatre, but many intensive care units now use techniques such as intermittent mandatory ventilation (IMV) and mandatory minute ventilation (MMV).

> Modes of ventilatory support include intermittent mandatory ventilation (IMV) and mandatory minute ventilation (MMV), more specialized techniques using high frequencies, and methods of improving oxygenation that apply end-expiratory pressure.

Although the abbreviations IMV and MMV are in common use, you must define them. The essay *must* start with full ventilation and its variants.

Full ventilatory support
>   set tidal volume and rate
>   for: simple
>   against: need for sedation (and paralysis)
>   uses: perioperative
>   ITU before any recovery
>   patient-initiated
>   for: patients settle better
>   against: may be inappropriate ventilation

Concentrate on ventilation in the intensive care unit, but for completeness you should mention routine intraoperative ventilation. Discuss the likely settings of tidal volume and rate; do not discuss the drugs you might use for sedation. Explain the principle behind the assisting of a patient's ventilation, and write a sentence or two about the workings of a specific ventilator, if you know about one. Do not abbreviate full ventilatory support to FMV; on repetition write of 'full ventilation'.

Partial support
>   by intermittent breaths (IMV)
>   by preset volume (MMV)
>   by assisting

For each of these you must write a description and give the advantages and disadvantages. The two sections you have now completed should be about two-thirds of the essay, and the rest will be shorter comments about techniques that are less common or that are less easily defined as support of ventilation.

Negative pressure ventilation

iron lung, cuirass, rocking bed

Prolonged mechanical ventilation dates from the epidemics of poliomyelitis in the 1950s, and a full answer includes the historical perspective.

Other forms of ventilation

independent lung
high frequency
variations of intra-cycle pressure and flow

This last list is of techniques aimed mainly at improving oxygenation rather than ventilation, but high frequency techniques have a place when ventilation is difficult (for instance if there is a large bronchopleural fistula or when compliance is very low). For Part 1 FCAnaes, these techniques are irrelevant; for Part 3, candidates will be expected to know something of them although, as there are almost as many modes of application as enthusiasts for them, candidates should concentrate on the principles rather than the precise details of tidal volumes and rates.

7-2 Discuss the methods available for sedation of patients undergoing mechanical ventilation in the intensive care unit.

OUTLINE PLAN

Sedation score

Before drugs
reassurance
adjust ventilation
general comfort

Opioid analgesics
some examples
side-effects

Non-opioids

Sedatives
midazolam
chlormethiazole

Intravenous anaesthetics
propofol
(barbiturates)

Inhalational agents
nitrous oxide, isoflurane

Neuromuscular relaxants

Possible opening sentences:

> Amongst the types of drug used commonly in the intensive care unit to sedate patients are narcotic analgesics, benzodiazepines, and intravenous anaesthetics.

> Patients can be treated on intensive care units without sedation but this ideal is not always possible.

> There is no need for patients to be rendered totally unconscious during their stay in the intensive care unit.

The better sentences are those that tell the examiner immediately that sedation is not essential. A settled patient *is* essential, and for that reason neuromuscular relaxants are sometimes necessary. It may be better to leave this for later in the answer, instead of listing relaxants in the opening sentence.

Sedation is difficult to measure, but you need some sort of definition; this one is attributed to Ramsay and colleagues.

Level of sedation
1. anxious, agitated, restless
2. cooperative, oriented, tranquil
3. responds to commands only
4. asleep, brisk response to glabellar tap or loud sound
5. asleep, sluggish response
6. no response

Aim: 2–4

Before discussing drugs, discuss methods of settling the patient and making them comfortable and able to accept their surroundings.

Reassurance

Ventilation
synchronize
moderate hypocapnia, large tidal volume

General comfort
nasotracheal tube, nasogastric tube, pressure areas
use of local anaesthesia

Unavoidable hypoxia, which is hypoxia caused by the condition, is a common reason for needing to give sedation. Anaesthetists do not aim for normoxia as a way of avoiding the need for sedation, so avoidance of hypoxia is not in this list.

When discussing specific drugs under their headings, choose drugs with which you are familiar.

Opioid analgesics

    the most commonly used drugs: for pain and to
        depress ventilatory drive
  morphine (but renal excretion)
  fentanyl (but false reputation for short duration)
  phenoperidine (potent, liked by some, cardiovascular
    stability)

Side-effects

  ventilatory depression
  hypotension
  gastrointestinal motility
  tolerance

The opioids are given to reduce ventilatory drive, and the reduction becomes a side effect only during weaning or if the ventilator fails or becomes disconnected. This needs to be stated explicitly. It is amazing how many candidates write 'A disadvantage of using opioids is that they reduce drive' without making these qualifications, thus contradicting the very reason for which they claim they are using the drugs.

Tolerance, the need for increasing doses, is more of a problem than addiction; but addiction can cause difficulties occasionally during weaning.

Non-opioid

  indomethacin suppositories: arthritic or bone pain
  epidurals

Arthritis does not go away because an elderly patient is on the intensive care unit with a more serious condition, and opioids are ineffective at relieving painful joints.

Sedatives

  benzodiazepines
    sedation, amnesia, muscle relaxation
    mild cardiovascular and ventilatory effects
      midazolam: commonest because no active
        metabolites, short (2–4 hours) elimination
        half-life (?in seriously ill)
      flumazenil to reverse
  chlormethiazole
    anticonvulsant
    use: acute confusional state, delirium tremens
    problem: large volumes, cumulation

Chlormethiazole is used much less commonly than midazolam because it is unusual that patients requiring intensive care can tolerate such large fluid loads. It does not, therefore, require much detail or discussion.

Intravenous anaesthetics

propofol
  advantages
    short elimination half-life, easily adjustable sedation
    does not suppress plasma cortisol
      (cf. etomidate)
  disadvantages
    cardiovascular depression
    loading, maintenance
    expensive
Barbiturates: prolonged recovery, mainly head injury

The question asks about sedation for *ventilation*. It is worth mentioning the use of thiopentone for cerebral protection in head injuries but there is no need for any detail of this contentious subject. Etomidate should be mentioned only in passing.

Inhalational anaesthetic agents

nitrous oxide: megaloblastic bone marrow changes
isoflurane: little biotransformation, under study

Neuromuscular relaxants

last resort (but disconnection!)
  never alone
atracurium infusion best (laudanosine irrelevant)

Relaxants are sometimes used when there are not enough nurses to look after all the patients. This is expedient: without doubt there are many patients who have been prevented from extubating themselves by a judicious dose of pancuronium. However, this is unacceptable medical practice and not for writing about in the FCAnaes.

7-3 Discuss the indications and advantages of positive end-expiratory pressure during mechanical ventilation. What are the harmful effects of this technique and how may they be minimized?

OUTLINE PLAN

Indications

prophylactic
therapeutic

threshold oxygenation
'best' PEEP

Mechanism

increasing functional residual capacity
reducing water and protein flux into alveoli

Harmful effects

on lung
cardiovascular
renal
neurological

Assessing and controlling PEEP

watch blood pressure
   measure cardiac output
maintain circulating volume
care with certain patients

This looks an easy question, but think about the subject for a moment or two and it becomes clear that there is really only one indication: hypoxia unrelieved by increasing the inspired concentration of oxygen; and what exactly is meant by 'advantages'? The advantages of being less hypoxic are self-evident and the only other advantage is that PEEP may help avoid oxygen toxicity — if you believe oxygen toxicity is a problem in these patients, and some do not.

The opening sentence gives the opportunity to define the abbreviation PEEP, which is now standard. It is difficult to think of any way of starting this answer other than with the words 'Positive end-expiratory pressure (PEEP) . . .'.

> Positive end-expiratory pressure (PEEP) is often used for hypoxic patients who require mechanical ventilation in the intensive care unit.

> Positive end-expiratory pressure (PEEP) is used to improve oxygenation in patients who have adult respiratory distress syndrome.

> Positive end-expiratory pressure (PEEP) increases the arterial partial pressure of oxygen (PaO_2) at a given inspired oxygen, but at the cost of reducing cardiac output by decreasing venous return.

The first sentence is too weak; it does little more than restate the question. The second is too specific; there are other indications besides adult respiratory distress syndrome. The third sentence is the best, providing a brief answer to the whole question.

Indications

prophylactic

to prevent atelectasis: 1–5 cm H_2O
therapeutic
to improve oxygenation: 6–20 cmH_2O
threshold PaO_2 less than 8 kPa on 50-60% oxygen
'best' PEEP

It is unusual these days for any ventilated patient in intensive care *not* to be given a few centimetres of PEEP. There is, however, little evidence that prophylactic PEEP is of benefit (it is of no benefit in fit healthy patients undergoing routine general anaesthesia) and you must be prepared in Part 3 FCAnaes to discuss this.

You must explain why the oxygenation threshold is 8 kPa and why the preferred inspired oxygen concentration is no higher than 60%.

You can define 'best' PEEP at this stage, but full discussion might be better left until the section on cardiovascular consequences.

Although the question does not ask directly, you need to discuss how PEEP is thought to work:

Mechanism

increasing functional residual capacity
preventing water and protein flux into alveoli
improved surfactant function
release of prostaglandins from lung tissue

There is no doubt that functional residual capacity increases and that, by hydrostatic forces, alveoli can be made less wet. The other suggested mechanisms, and more may emerge, are less clear. Do not put forward assertive quasi-scientific explanations. There are many things in medicine that we know work but for which we have imperfect explanations (the mode of action of general anaesthetics being one) and there is nothing wrong with admitting thoughtful ignorance.

Harmful effects

on lung
    barotrauma
    increased shunt
cardiovascular
    decreased venous return
    increased pulmonary vascular resistance
renal
    decreased renal blood flow
neurological
    increased intracranial pressure

The basic rule for minimizing these effects is to keep the intrathoracic pressure as low as possible, in other words to limit PEEP to only what is deemed necessary.

Assessing and controlling PEEP

watch blood pressure
  measure cardiac output
  monitor mixed venous oxygen saturation
maintain circulating volume
dopamine for renal blood flow?
care with certain patients
  intracranial pressure
  abnormal lungs etc.

Do not suggest that 'best' PEEP can be applied only if there are frequent measurements of cardiac output and continuous measurement of venous saturation. In someone who needs high levels of PEEP to maintain oxygenation it is clinically obvious from the subsequent hypotension that the heart is compromised.

Dopamine is commonly used, but there is as yet no clear evidence that it protects against acute renal failure. This is a good topic for discussion.

PEEP may be better avoided in some patients, for example those with emphysematous bullae or with pneumothorax. Note that the question does not ask about continuous positive airways pressure (CPAP).

7-4 What are the factors affecting the ability to wean patients from ventilators? Discuss the criteria and methods used for weaning patients from ventilatory support.

OUTLINE PLAN

Factors affecting weaning

the initial disease
systems
  respiratory
  other
effects of treatment
psychological

Criteria

keep factors in mind
mechanical pulmonary function
gas exchange

Methods

stop drugs
techniques
  T piece, more sophisticated circuitry
    descriptions, advantages, disadvantages
assessment

This is a 'bread-and-butter' question in intensive care; no matter what the disease, the same conditions have to be met before these steps on the way to full recovery can be taken. The question is also a good differentiator between candidates who have read the books and those who have practical experience. It is a question that allows you to write your own opinions; despite the large number of techniques advocated at one time or another, most patients can be weaned successfully — though it might take longer and require more attention from the nurses and anaesthetists — simply by allowing them intermittently to breathe spontaneously until they are clinically satisfactory.

Opening sentences can be simply factual or can be used to give an opinion.

> A patient should be weaned from the ventilator once the underlying problems that necessitated ventilation are resolving.

> There are many techniques for weaning patients from ventilators, and the personal preferences of the clinicians often govern practice in each intensive care unit.

> The approach when considering any patient for weaning consists of the questions: Are they ready?; Can they manage?; How quickly will they wean?; Was it successful?

The structure of the question gives the basic structure of the answer: start with the factors to consider before contemplating weaning.

Factors affecting weaning
  the initial disease
    infection
  systems
    respiratory
      oxygenation
      ventilation
        $PaCO_2$, muscles, effusion, pneumothorax
    cardiac
    renal
    intestinal and feeding
    neurological
  effects of treatment
    drugs
  psychological
  fear and dependence, pain, sleep deprivation

Most of this can be summed up by saying that successful weaning is unlikely if the patient's original disease is still active, or if there is infection, severe catabolism, and failure of one or more organs — in addition to the lungs.

Do not be too repetitive when discussing respiratory factors considered *before* weaning and the criteria used *during* weaning. The advantage of writing an essay plan is that you then know that you will return to a subject later and so can write '(see below)'. There should be different emphasis in the two sections. While the patient is being ventilated, the partial pressures of the arterial gases allow a quick assessment of 'Are they ready?'; the mechanical considerations of 'Can they manage?' apply to spontaneous ventilation.

Criteria

  keep factors (as above) in mind
    haemodynamic
  mechanical pulmonary function
    vital capacity more than 10–15 ml/kg
    tidal volume more than 5 ml/kg
    peak inspiratory pressure greater than –20 cm H_2O
    resting minute volume more than 10 L/min
  gas exchange
    PaO_2 at least 8 kPa on 40% oxygen
    $D(A–a)O_2$ less than 40 kPa on 100% oxygen
    dead space ratio less than 0.6

Weaning can cause marked haemodynamic changes and these need some discussion.

You need to give some figures — and anyone who has read the books can do that. We have given some here. They may differ from the figures you know or that you use on your ICU. We have put the values in, not because they are correct (you should not be learning numbers from this book), but to introduce some discussion. If you look in different textbooks you will find different numbers. Some are widely accepted and based on sound physiological principles (a PaO_2 of 8 kPa is above the steep part of the oxyhaemoglobin dissociation curve); others are based on clinical experience and show wide variability between patients. As so often for the examinations, it is clinical experience that is most important, as it is when making practical clinical decisions about weaning.

Those with experience of the intensive care unit will know that measures of mechanical function are not usually made, nor is it usual to calculate the dead space ratio; it is this sort of comment that enables examiners to tell who is writing from experience. However, beware being deprecatory and blasé about the measurements. The correct approach is not 'You can do these tests, but frankly why bother?' but 'These are the tests which, although not always applied, can be useful.'

Methods

  sedative drugs, time of day
  techniques

      T piece
          continuous/intermittent
          advantages: simple
          disadvantages: needs attention
            may be slower
    IMV, SIMV, MMV, inspiratory support
      describe
          advantages: probably more pleasant for patient
           easier for attendants
           may be quicker
    CPAP

Assessment

You must give firm statements of what you do about the various sedatives, opioids, and muscle relaxants the patient might be on. In practice, weaning is usually started early in the day to allow the full working day in which to judge its success. As all the techniques have the same supposed advantages, it saves time to describe them as a group and then discuss the advantages of the group. The abbreviations are all standard and anyone taking Part 3 should be familiar with them. They should nonetheless be defined when first written. CPAP is kept separate because it is not a ventilatory support but a method for maintaining the PaO_2.

7-5   <u>Discuss the diagnosis of brain death.</u>

OUTLINE PLAN

Preconditions

    brain damage, coma, drugs, metabolism

Testing

    cranial nerves
    ventilation

Personnel

(Other investigations)

Remaining problems

The following is a good solid opening sentence, which also allows the abbreviation EEG to be defined. It forms a good introduction to an essay in which the conditions for diagnosis can be enumerated and described — and that is probably what the examiners want.

> Brain stem death is now considered to be a definition of death itself because cardiac asystole with an isoelectric electroencephalogram (EEG) has always followed brain stem death within a few days.

There are other approaches to this question though, for example that of the philosopher or ethicist, or that of the medical historian. We would not advise these approaches in an essay, although you could try them in a viva (the examiners would soon stop you if what they wished to know was just a list of the criteria). These other approaches would give excellent opening sentences for Part 3, though they are probably inappropriate at Part 1:

> The diagnosis of brain death became necessary when it became possible to support virtually indefinitely the cardiorespiratory function of patients with irreversible brain damage.

> There is a public misconception that brain death was invented so that organs could be taken for transplants, but the concept would be needed even if transplantation was impossible.

> Until recently, the outward sign of death was cessation of the heart beat, but modern technology has rendered this definition obsolete.

If you use an opening sentence of this type, do not be distracted for too long from the main substance:

Preconditions
    irremediable structural brain damage
        known diagnosis
    apnoeic coma
    drugs
        history, investigations
    metabolism
        no gross disturbance
        normothermic

The preconditions are important, so give some detail and some examples.

Testing
    cranial nerves
        pupils
        eyelash, corneal reflexes
        facial pain response
        caloric reflex
        gag, carinal reflexes
    ventilation
        hyperoxic
        increase PaCO$_2$

The complete answer must include full descriptions of how you perform these tests.

Personnel
two doctors
not of transplant team
perform tests twice

(Other investigations
EEG and carotid angiography)

Remaining problems
not unanimity
beating-heart donors

The sections on other investigations and remaining problems would not be needed for Part 1, where it is the mechanics of the how, why and who of testing that is important. The Part 3 candidate must be aware that not everyone has the same view of brain death, and that there are some who disapprove of taking organs from a donor whose heart is still beating. 'Other investigations' is in brackets to indicate that these tests should be mentioned only briefly; they are not necessary in Britain.

7-6 Discuss the intensive care management of a patient with Guillain–Barré syndrome (acute postinfective polyneuritis).

OUTLINE PLAN

Ventilatory support
assessment, ETT or tracheostomy?, ventilation
physiotherapy

Autonomic assessment

Monitoring
before decision to ventilate
during ventilation

Treatment
definitive
supportive
other

Recovery
timing, extubation?, discharge?

The question asks for the intensive care management, so you can assume that the diagnosis has been made. You should plan the answer from the neurologist's request that the patient be admitted through to the stage of recovery that allows the patient to be discharged to the general ward.

Not all patients with Guillain–Barré syndrome will require

mechanical ventilation, but if they do they may need ventilating for several weeks.

Patients with Guillain–Barré syndrome may require ventilating if they develop ventilatory failure or bulbar palsy.

Guillain–Barré affects motor, sensory, and autonomic function.

These are all general opening sentences; none is outstanding but all are satisfactory. You could start with a definition of the syndrome, but that would probably merely repeat the parenthesis in the question. Do not use any abbreviation (GBS or APN or whatever). Comparing the first and second sentences, 'Patients may require mechanical ventilation' is better than 'Patients may require ventilating'.

Note that patients with the syndrome develop *ventilatory* failure, which is specifically failure to ventilate the lungs, and not *respiratory* failure, which may include ventilatory failure by common usage but is better used when there is failure of gas exchange at the alveolar membrane.

There is no need to discuss differential diagnosis, and the first section of the answer should centre on the decision to ventilate.

Ventilatory support
 assessment of ventilatory failure
 assessment of bulbar palsy
 nasotracheal tube versus early tracheostomy
  ventilator settings
 physiotherapy

At Part 3, you will be expected to know the arguments in favour of the two options for the airway. Do not go into automatic answering mode when writing about the settings of the ventilator: unlike most patients who are being ventilated on the ICU, patients with Guillain–Barré are likely to be fully conscious and to have healthy lungs (at least to start with).

Monitoring
 before decision to ventilate
 during intubation
  autonomic disturbances
 during ventilation
  ventilatory
  cardiovascular
  other

Treatment
 definitive
  corticosteroids, cytotoxics
  plasmapheresis

Details of definitive treatments, all of which are somewhat empirical and experimental, will not be expected at Part 1. Autonomic disturbances can be life-threatening and perhaps even warrant a separate paragraph before the section on ventilatory support.

> supportive
> > fluids and electrolytes, feeding
> > urinary catheter
> > care of eyes
> > limb physiotherapy
> > psychological

Psychological support is always needed for patients who are conscious while being treated in the ICU; it is an important part of this answer. The best support for patients with Guillain–Barré, who fear they will never recover from their paralysis, is counselling from patients who have themselves recovered from the condition.

> other
> > chest infections
> > sedation
> > muscle cramps
> > DVT prophylaxis

Chest infections will need most discussion in this section.

> **Recovery**
> > timing, prognostic signs
> > decision to extubate
> > decision to discharge to ward

Your answer ends with discharge to the general ward. Late recovery is not part of the intensive care management.

7-7   Discuss the management of a patient admitted to the intensive care unit with acute severe asthma.

OUTLINE PLAN

Features

Management
> investigations
> immediate treatment: general, specific, other

Reassessment
> ventilation
> > suggestions and problems
> when improving

The opening sentence should define what is meant by acute severe asthma.

Acute severe asthma is a life-threatening asthmatic attack that is resistant to conventional therapy.

It should be followed by a list of clinical features and the expected results of immediate investigations. There is no need for any discussion of the aetiology or pathology of asthma except perhaps when justifying particular treatments; nor for descriptions of the more usual presentations of the disease. The question is quite clear. You are not being asked how to assess whether a patient needs to be admitted to the unit; the patient has been admitted and you are being asked for your management.

Features
extreme dyspnoea — no speech
poor air entry — 'silent chest'
central cyanosis — $\dot{V}/\dot{Q}$ mismatch
tachycardia: pulse rate > 130/min
pulsus paradoxus
hypercapnia
impaired conscious level

Management
establish diagnosis
establish intravenous access, sample
  full blood count
  urea and electrolytes
sputum sample
insert arterial line, sample
chest X-ray
spirometry if possible

Although the patient has already been admitted, and you do not have to give details about initial diagnosis, it is worth putting in a sentence to the effect that you need to be sure of the diagnosis.

Everyone knows about pulsus paradoxus, though it is not particularly useful clinically, even in less severe asthma, now that arterial gas tensions and pulse oximetry are so readily available.

For each investigation, you must write what you expect to find. Patients in the early stages of an attack are hypocapnic but this patient will be at best normocapnic. Do not forget acid–base balance in your discussion of the arterial sample.

Treatment
  humidified oxygen
  adequate hydration
drugs

> nebulized salbutamol
> ipratropium bromide
> adrenaline
> aminophylline
> antibiotics
> steroids
> sedation
> physiotherapy

General treatment should always come before specific treatment; and immediate treatment before later treatment. Some treatments are contentious; for instance, some believe not merely that aminophylline is not a good drug for relieving bronchospasm but that its cardiac effects make it dangerous. You will be expected to know appropriate doses of the bronchodilators. It is best to avoid sedation, but the judicious use of benzodiazepines combined with reassurance can be helpful.

Then

> assess
> if worse (hypercapnia, exhaustion, mental state)
>   consider ventilation
> large tidal volume, slow rate
> no PEEP
> sufficient sedation
> bronchoscopy, lavage
> care: barotrauma, right ventricular failure
> extubation: cover by anaesthesia

A final comment might be that because asthma can be unpredictable, it is worth visiting the ward once or twice after the patient has been discharged from the unit.

7-8   Discuss the management during the first 48 hours of an adult patient with a severe burn.

OUTLINE PLAN

Immediate action

Assessment of burn

Early analgesia

Fluids

> where, what, assessment

Inhalational injury

> recognition and treatment

Definitive treatment
infection control, dressings, surgery

Other treatment
analgesia, metabolic support

Complications

This is a very general question, from which it is all too easy to miss important headings. Questions have been asked on the restricted topic of the management of just the pulmonary complications of burns (see next page).

The immediate problems from a severe burn are hypovolaemia from loss of plasma, and the pulmonary complications of inhalation of poisonous or hot gases.

The anaesthetist's involvement with the severely burned patient usually starts after the patient has been admitted to hospital.

Severely burned patients are often surprisingly well when first admitted to hospital, but treatment must be rapid and well organized for the patient to have the best chance of avoiding the many life-threatening complications.

The management obviously starts with removing the patient from the fire, and giving necessary treatment at the site. Any of these three opening sentences is good; the last two define hospital as the starting point for treatment, and for your answer.

Immediately
circulation, breathing, conscious level, reassurance

Assessment of burn
depth
surface area

There are a number of formulae, the rule of nine being the most common but not the only one. The question asks about adults; do not make any mention of children.

Reassurance is mentioned specifically. Some patients admitted to hospital with serious diseases do not realize just how ill they are; severe burns are known to be dangerous and patients are almost always anxious.

Early analgesia

Fluids
intravenous site(s)
type and volume
monitoring
clinical, urine, investigations
difficulties

Be confident about the types and volumes of fluid. Do not give the examiner the impression that you always give fluid according to a formula, no matter which authority you can quote. The more seriously burned the patient, the less useful are the formulae as anything more than rough guidelines for treating individuals: the most important emphasis is on the need for frequent reassessment.

'Difficulties' are with monitoring and intravenous cannulation. Where would you place a pulse oximeter probe on a patient with burned hands, feet and ears?

Inhalational injury
carbon monoxide, burn, toxic fumes
recognition and treatment

Definitive treatment
infection
isolation, topical antibiotics
surgery
dressing, early grafts

Other treatment
continuing analgesia
metabolic support

Complications
renal failure
stress ulcer
electrolyte disturbance

The question is about the first 48 hours. Discussion about renal failure and stress ulcers should be confined to how best to prevent them by the institution of early treatment. The use of suxamethonium is not contra-indicated in the first 48 hours. The problem of repeated anaesthetics for burns dressing is also a later problem.

7-9 Discuss the intensive care management of respiratory complications in patients with major burns.

OUTLINE PLAN

Carbon monoxide poisoning
oxyhaemoglobin dissociation curve;
diagnosis: history, symptoms and signs, investigations
treatment: 100% oxygen, hyperbaric
outcome: neurological

Inhalation of toxic fumes
types and effects

> diagnosis
> treatment
> oedema, ARDS, pulmonary infection

Thermal injury
> heat and oedema
> diagnosis: appearance, stridor, look
> treatment: ? intubation (early)

Best is a simple, direct opening sentence that gives the headings and structure of the answer.

> Major burns have three main respiratory complications: carbon monoxide poisoning; the inhalation of toxic fumes; and thermal injury to the respiratory tract.

The answer is now a matter of working through each of these subjects, spending about the same amount of time on each. Within each subject, a useful rough outline is 'definition — effect — diagnosis — treatment — outcome'. If you use the abbreviation CO for carbon monoxide, do not use it also for cardiac output, and make your writing clear so there is no confusion with CO_2.

Carbon monoxide poisoning
> when carboxyhaemoglobin (HbCO) exceeds 20%
> effect: on oxyhaemoglobin dissociation curve (diag)
> on cytochrome oxidase
> diagnosis
> history
> symptoms and signs related to % of HbCO
> investigations: blood gases
> co-oximetry
> treatment: 100% oxygen
> ventilation
> hyperbaric chamber
> outcome: neurological

The best way to describe what happens to the oxyhaemoglobin dissociation curve is to draw it. You can then write: 'The diagram shows the effect of carbon monoxide on the curve, and the physiological result is . . .'

There is no need to include any details for ventilation; there is nothing special about the way the patient is ventilated just because of carbon monoxide poisoning. However, there are few indications for using a hyperbaric chamber, so you should write something about the way it would be used, and discuss briefly the advantages and disadvantages.

Inhalation of toxic fumes
> carbonaceous material, acids, cyanide

```
        oedema of airways
        specific effects
    diagnosis
        history
    treatment
        of airway oedema
        of adult respiratory distress syndrome (ARDS)
        of pulmonary infection
```

The history — which means, 'What was burning?' — is extremely important in burns, as there are not necessarily any specific symptoms and signs. It is not widely known that burning foam furniture gives off cyanides. These can reach high enough concentrations in the victims to poison rescuers doing mouth-to-airway resuscitation.

Thermal injury is the main cause of airway oedema. On our plan, thermal injury is the next section but airway oedema has already been introduced. There is no time for repetition when writing examination answers, so write '(see below)'. The treatment of ARDS is a question in itself; give no more than the barest outline here.

Thermal injury

```
        heat
            oedema
        diagnosis
            appearance: facial, mucosal, sputum
            stridor
        treatment
            ?intubation (early)
```

Heat can damage tissue without needing smoke and flames, but the airway is unlikely to be damaged if there are no facial signs. Thermal injury is of the large airways. Writing '?intubation (early)' in the plan indicates not that this is the best treatment, but that you should include discussion of the factors you would consider. It is not the burn itself, or the respiratory effects, that are the problem; it is that intubation may become very difficult, and is best attempted with as little haste as possible.

There is nothing specific to put for outcome after thermal injury.

There are two general points to make about this question. The wording is 'respiratory complications', which must include the physiological effects of carbon monoxide and cyanide as well as the physical effects of acid fumes and heat. If the question had asked for *pulmonary complications* then the meaning would not be clear, because carbon monoxide and cyanide have no effect on the lung. If faced with a problem of interpretation, ask the examiner, and then, if still in doubt, define your interpretation in your first paragraph.

Discussion of the rule of nine, or any other aspect of burns, is not relevant to this question.

7-10 Outline the principles of control of cross-infection in the intensive care unit.

OUTLINE PLAN

Personal hygiene

Invasive procedures

Equipment

Antibiotics

involve microbiologist

Organization

Opening sentence:

Cross-infection in the intensive care unit can delay recovery of the patients or even threaten their lives.

Cross-infection in the intensive care unit (ICU) is a complication of 30–40% of admissions.

Hospital-acquired infections can complicate any admission and they are even more likely in the intensive care unit (ICU) where the patients are debilitated, there is frequent close contact between patients and staff, and invasive procedures are a normal part of treatment.

The first sentence is weak; the same is true of any infection acquired in hospital. The second shows you know it is a serious problem. The third is the best because it leads into the structure of the answer.

Routes and organisms

other patients (direct/indirect), staff
air-borne, contact, ingestion
increased likelihood of infection

General control: within patient, of contact

This first section gives a general introduction; mention the most common cross-infecting organisms, where they come from (not forgetting that the ward itself can be growing colonies of bacteria in rarely cleaned corners), and why patients on ICU are especially susceptible.

Your description should proceed logically; we keep repeating this advice because it is so important if you are aiming for a well structured answer that misses out nothing of importance: here that means you start by writing, 'Wash your hands . . .'.

Personal hygiene

Invasive procedures

  aseptic technique

  life of intravenous, intra-arterial, central venous lines

    care, choice of site

Equipment

  ventilators

    filters, maintenance

  humidifiers

  disposables

Antibiotics

  <u>involve microbiologist</u>

  take samples

  ?prophylaxis

    ?selective decontamination

Organization

  adequate separation of beds

  isolation

This whole plan flows nicely from one sub-heading to the next. Think about which topics in these lists and sub-lists you wish to stress; to some extent you have the luxury in this rather general essay to concentrate on topics of particular interest to you. If you have read recently about the benefit of using airway filters, or your hospital has been involved in a study of selective decontamination, then you have the opportunity to tell the examiners something they may not themselves know. Having said that, all headings and sub-headings need some expansion: 'isolation', for example, needs a comment about the types of patients, the types of infection and the way the ward will be organized. While all answers must include these comments, not everyone may know about the details of air changes and ventilation of isolation rooms.

The reference to the microbiology department is underlined due to its importance; examiners will certainly be looking for this in your answer.

Cross-infection in the context of this question means infection passing between patients and does not include the overt infection of staff with, for example, hepatitis and AIDS. Less certain is whether the answer should include reference to infection from transfused blood.

7-11 Discuss the differential diagnosis and management of stridor in a child aged 3 years.

OUTLINE PLAN

Definition and description of stridor

  mimicking conditions

true differential diagnosis

Acute epiglottitis

cause

clinical features

initial management

in the operating theatre

especially intubation

in the intensive care unit

especially when to extubate

Laryngotracheobronchitis

headings as for epiglottitis

Other conditions

enlarged tonsils

retropharyngeal abscess

subglottic stenosis

Foreign body

A stock Part 3 question. The most threatening diagnosis is acute epiglottitis, and a detailed description of its recognition and management is the main part of the answer. It is not clear from the question if the examiners want to know only about treating stridor, that is, the initial treatment of the child, or whether the answer should cover the whole course of the condition giving rise to the symptom. We suggest that discussion of the whole course is safer unless a question asks, 'Discuss the initial management of . . .'; an important point of management is when to remove a tracheal tube, and that must be discussed for a full answer to the question here.

Opening sentences:

Stridor is the cardinal sign of incomplete upper respiratory tract obstruction.

The best known diagnosis to cause stridor is acute epiglottitis, a life-threatening condition that can kill a child with alarming rapidity.

Stridor in a 3-year-old child is acute epiglottitis until proved otherwise.

This is not a difficult question for which to write an opening sentence; any of the above is good, and there are others that one can think of without having to try too hard. The plan must start with a description of stridor, which is not simply noisy breathing. However, discuss only conditions that cause stridor; bronchospasm, for example, should be mentioned as a differential diagnosis, but then dismissed for the purposes of your answer to this question.

Definition and description of stridor

 mimicking conditions
 true differential diagnosis
  pharyngeal
  laryngeal
  tracheal

There are many rare conditions that cause stridor, but the principles of initial management are the same because of the overriding worry that loss of the airway can occur suddenly and unexpectedly. Deal now with acute epiglottitis; if you show the examiner you understand these principles it matters less if you are not so certain in your differential diagnosis.

Acute epiglottitis

 cause
 clinical features
 initial management
  position
  antibiotics
 in the operating theatre
  surgeon
  drugs
  intubation

You must give a full description of an inhalational induction, the expected appearance at laryngoscopy, how you identify the larynx, what tracheal tube you use and how you secure it.

 in the intensive care unit
  continuing treatment
  assessment
  when to extubate

The main differential diagnosis is laryngotracheobronchitis and associated conditions, generally known as croup. They are less likely to progress as suddenly as epiglottitis, and the indications for intubation are more the standard ones of hypoxia and exhaustion. Croup can be discussed under parallel headings to those of epiglottitis, but remembering that specific treatment differs. In particular, bronchodilators may help.

Other conditions

 enlarged tonsils
 retropharyngeal abscess
 subglottic stenosis
  brief note on diagnosis and treatment for each

Foreign body

 larynx

trachea
bronchus

A bronchial foreign body does not cause stridor, although it should be considered in the initial differential diagnosis of a child with breathing difficulties. There is no need for more than simple statements about paediatric bronchoscopy.

7-12 What can be measured or derived from a successfully placed multilumen flow-directed pulmonary artery catheter?

This is a very difficult question. It gives no clue to what the examiners want to know. As it is written, candidates could simply give a list of all the variables it is possible to measure or derive. There is nothing in the question to suggest that the answer should even include the normal values, let alone interpretations of haemodynamic state or possible treatments. All sorts of calculations *can* be made from the measurements, but we do not know which is, or are, the most valuable. The humble systolic blood pressure is an index of myocardial contractility, and cardiovascular physiologists can argue for hours about other indices such as left ventricular stroke work index or rate of rise of arterial pressure, or countless others that each have their proponents.

Remember that there is still argument simply about the value of flow-directed pulmonary artery catheters.

Part of the skill of taking examinations is knowing which questions to omit (if there is a choice!), and this might be one to consider omitting.

Index to writing answers

Index to anaesthetic and medical terms